Health&Fitness MAGAZINE

TONE UP
in 10 MINUTES

Cover photography Ian Derry
Photography Will Ireland, Hugh Threlfall, Danny Bird,
Gareth Sambidge, Maja Smend
Models Sophie Hellyer @ W Athletic, Tess Montgomery @ MOT
Clothing from a selection at Sweaty Betty (sweatybetty.com),
Nike (nike.com), Freddy (020 7836 5291) and Shockabsorber (shockabsorber.co.uk)
Ball and band (used in exercises) Davina range at argos.co.uk
Editor Mary Comber
Sub-editors John Murphy, Emma Morris, Margaret Bartlett
Art editors Lucy Pinto, Holly White, Victoria Hill
Design Christine Leech, Louise Browne
Words Antonia Kanczula, Peter Muir, Joanna Ebsworth, Sarah Ivory

MagBook Publisher Dharmesh Mistry
Digital Production Manager Nicky Baker
Operations Director Robin Ryan
MagBook Account Manager Katie Wood
MagBook Account Executive Emma D'Arcy
Managing Director of Advertising Julian Lloyd-Evans
Newstrade Director David Barker
Retail & Commercial Director Martin Belson
Publisher Nicola Bates
Group Publisher Russell Blackman
Group Managing Director Ian Westwood
Chief Operating Officer Brett Reynolds
Group Finance Director Ian Leggett
Chief Executive James Tye
Chairman Felix Dennis

MAG**BOOK**

The 'MagBook' brand is a trademark of Dennis Publishing Ltd, 30 Cleveland St,
London W1T 4JD. Company registered in England. All material © Dennis Publishing Ltd, licensed by Felden 2010, and may not be
reproduced in whole or part without the consent of the publishers.

Tone up in 10 minutes ISBN 1-907232-81-8

To license this product, contact Ornella Roccoletti on +44 (0) 20 7907 6134 or
e-mail ornella_roccoletti @dennis.co.uk

While every care was taken during the production of this MagBook, the publishers cannot be held responsible for the accuracy
of the information or any consequence arising from it. Dennis Publishing takes no responsibility for the companies advertising in
this Magbook. The paper used within this MagBook is produced from sustainable fibre,
manufactured by mills with a valid chain of custody. Printed at BGP.

The health and fitness information presented in this book is an educational
resource and is not intended as a substitute for medical advice.
Consult your doctor or healthcare professional before performing any of the exercises described in this book or any other
exercise programme, particularly if you are pregnant, or if you are elderly or have chronic or recurring medical conditions. Do
not attempt any of the exercises while under the influence of alcohol or drugs. Discontinue any exercise that causes you pain or
severe discomfort and consult a medical expert. Neither the author of the information nor the producer nor distributors of such
information make any warranty of any kind in regard to the content of the information presented in this book.

Spring all year round...

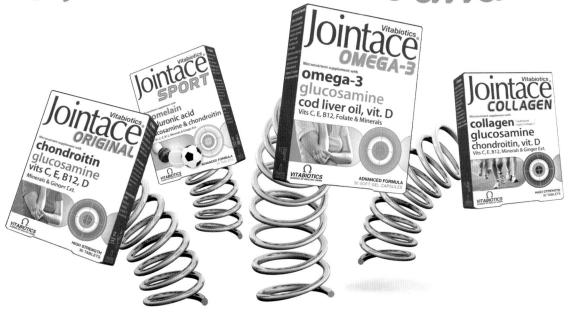

Cartilage and bone health are important for long term wellbeing and an active life. If you are looking for a daily supplement to give you extra support from within, *Jointace®* range has been specially formulated by Vitabiotics' experts to provide premium nutritional care. With a unique combination of nutrients, and vitamin C which contributes to normal collagen formation for the normal function of bone and cartilage.

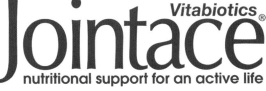

nutritional support for an active life

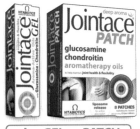

also GEL or PATCH
for direct application.
Ideal alongside *Jointace®* Tabs or Caps.

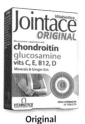

Original

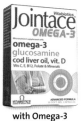

with Omega-3

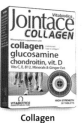

Collagen

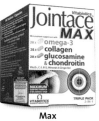

Max

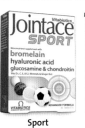

Sport

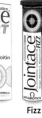

Fizz

From 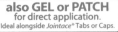, Superdrug, supermarkets, Lloydspharmacy, chemists, Holland & Barrett, GNC, health stores & *www.jointace.com*
Vitamin supplements may benefit those with nutritionally inadequate diets.

Voted Favourite
Supplement in its class
by Boots Customers

Most
loved
vitamins as
voted by you

Britain's leading supplements
for specific life stages

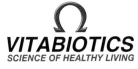
VITABIOTICS
SCIENCE OF HEALTHY LIVING

ADJONSPRINGP 13-02-13E

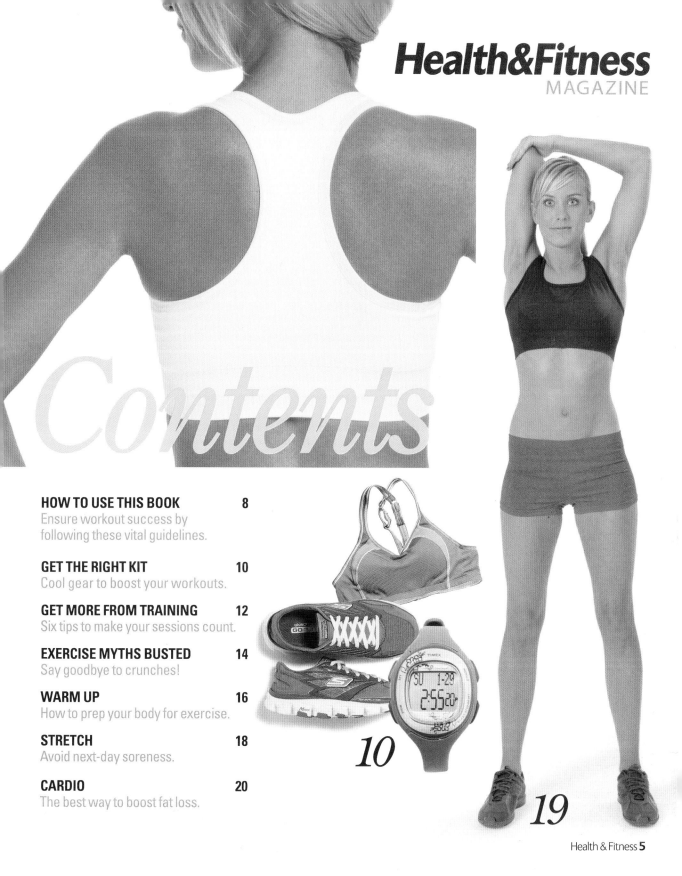

Health&Fitness
MAGAZINE

Contents

10

19

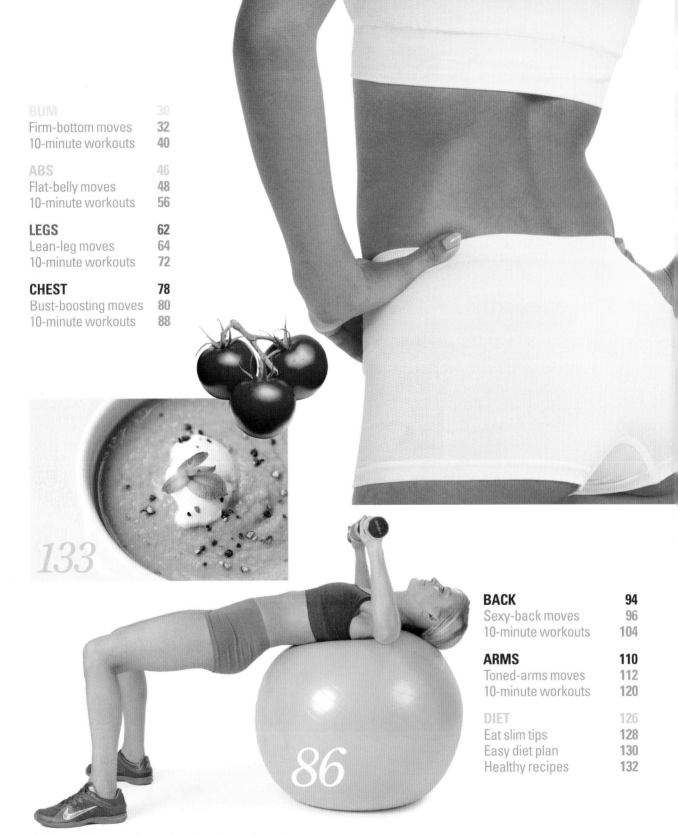

Look out for new cans in store

* * * * NEED A * * * *
NATURAL
LIFT?

contains fruit juice

Natural Energy Drink

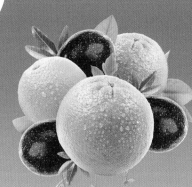

delicious
orange & passion fruit

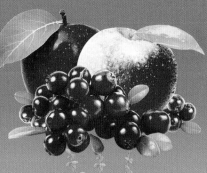

refreshing
cranberry & apple

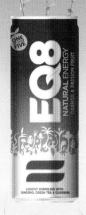

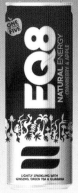

1 OF 5 YOUR A DAY

Available from* Morrisons, Sainsbury's and Tesco

eq8energy.com ★ facebook.com/eq8energy ★ twitter.com/eq8energy

*selected stores

EQ8
NATURAL ENERGY DRINK

HOW TO USE THIS BOOK

You're raring to go – but read these guidelines before you get started.

We know you're short on time, but we also know you want results and no-nonsense advice from your fitness plan. That's why we've created *Tone up in 10 minutes*, to help you achieve your dream body shape quickly, easily and safely. Doing a short workout three days a week, a cardio session on two days and resting on the remaining two days of the week, you can make regular, effective exercise a sustainable part of your life.

1 SCULPT AND TONE

The first part of this book is divided into six sections, one for each of your main body parts: bum, abdominals, legs, chest, back and arms. In each section, you'll find eight power exercises, expertly designed to tone up your trouble spots. These moves are effective, safe and straightforward – no complicated instructions! Use these to create your own workouts or follow the 10-minute circuits at the end of each section.

CHEST

The daily grind can really weaken your upper body. Driving a car and working at a computer constrict the chest muscles and lead to tension in the back. This set of exercises is designed to pep up your posture, open up your shoulders and tone up your pectorals and bust.

SIX WAYS TO A PERT BUST

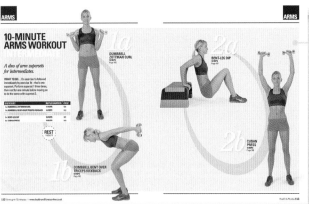

2 10-MINUTE CIRCUITS

Following the exercises in each section are three targeted tone-up circuits, rated beginner, intermediate and advanced. Each of these circuits contains a tailored mix of moves to blitz your trouble spot in 10 minutes. Aim to do three toning workouts a week. Choose the body part you want to target and the workout level that suits your fitness level.

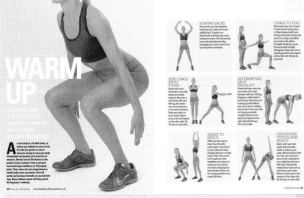

WARM UP

JUMPING JACKS
LUNGE TO FLYE
SIDE LUNGE WITH TWIST
ALTERNATING SPLIT DEADLIFT
SQUAT TO REACH
CROSSOVER TOUCH AND REACH

3 AVOID INJURY

Before each workout, remember to warm up and prepare your muscles, using the advice and moves on pages 16 and 17.

4 ... AND RELAX

Following your workout, take time to cool down and stretch your muscles. Our cool-down and stretching moves on page 18 will do the trick.

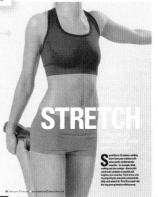

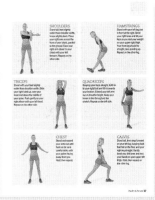

STRETCH

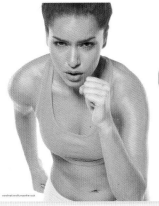

CARDIO

5 BOOST YOUR FITNESS

For maximum fat-burning effects, supplement your toning workouts with calorie-burning cardio sessions a week. Choose from our activity ideas on pages 22-23 and check out our simple chart to help you plan your days.

6 EAT SLIM!

This is a total body plan. To rev up your workout results, follow the healthy eating advice from page 132. As well as an easy seven-day diet plan, you'll find loads of tasty tips and ultra-lean recipes.

RECIPES

Rustling up tasty – and healthy – meals doesn't have to be a chore. These easy recipes have all the nutrients your hardworking body needs.

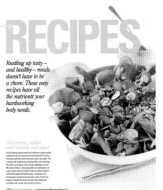

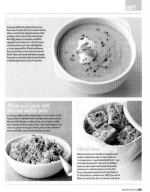

1

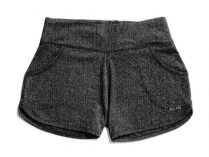

2

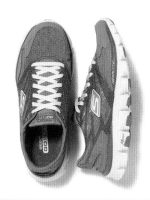

3

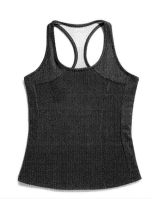

4

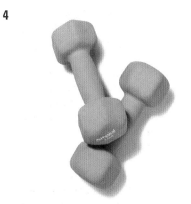

THE KIT

We've made the workouts as kit-light as possible, but there are a few essentials you shouldn't be without. You'll need a few pieces of gear, particularly as your fitness progresses, but there's no need to splash out on the latest high-tech innovations. Your kit list – a gym ball, mat, resistance band and dumbbells – can be just as effective.

5

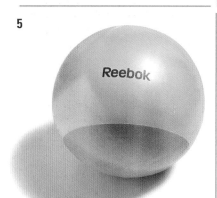
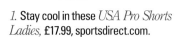

6

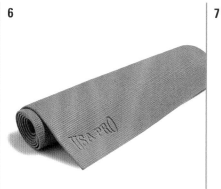

7

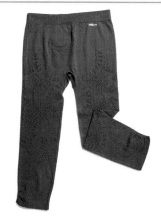

1. Stay cool in these *USA Pro Shorts Ladies,* £17.99, sportsdirect.com.

2. Boost your natural stride in *SKECHERS GOrun Ride,* £70, skechers.co.uk.

3. Increase your metabolic rate by 18% with the *Zaggora HoT Top,* £50, zaggora.com.

4. Build muscle with the *Neo-Hex Dumbell, 5kg,* £14.50, physicalcompany.co.uk.

5. Reebok Gym Ball – 65 cm, £29.99, reebokfitness.info – with instructional DVD.

6. USA Pro's Yoga Mat, £6.99, store. usapro.co.uk, has an anti-slip quilted surface.

7. adidas Women's Adipure Seamless ¾ Tights, £26, adidas.co.uk. Flat-waisted for comfort, with Climacool technology, these tights are perfect for any workout.

8. Stay warm and dry whatever the weather in the *Dounlimited Women's Performance Running Vest,* £35, dounlimited.com.

8

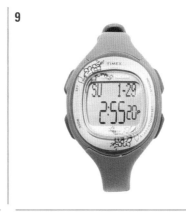

9

10

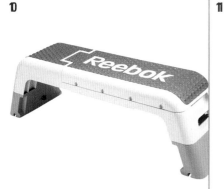

11

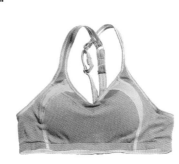

12

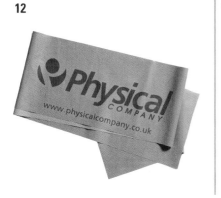

13

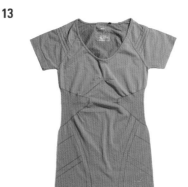

STAY SAFE!

◆ Always warm up properly to prepare your body and prevent injury.

◆ Listen to your body – don't exercise if you're unwell and stop immediately if you feel pain.

◆ Watch your form! Think quality over quantity. Perform each exercise with precision and engage your core muscles throughout to protect your back.

◆ Choose the correct dumbbell weight – one that's challenging but still allows you to perform all the prescribed repetitions (reps) for each exercise. If you're a novice, pick a weight you can manage easily the first time you perform any lifting exercise. Concentrate on performing the exercise perfectly, then build up the weight once you've mastered the move.

◆ Progress your workouts incrementally. Don't be tempted to do too much too soon. But at the same time, remember that your body adapts well to stress, so you should be regularly upping the intensity of your workouts.

◆ Rehydrate and refuel. Sip water during your workouts and always nourish your body afterwards with a snack that combines carbohydrates and protein, such as a peanut butter sandwich or recovery milkshake. Make sure you get muscle-replenishing nutrients into your body within 40 minutes after your workout.

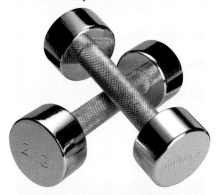

9. Timex Health Tracker, £59.99, timex.co. uk, will help you keep track of your progress.

10. Boost your weights sessions with the *Reebok Deck,* £199.99, reebokfitness.info.

11. Beat the bounce with the *Urban X-Over A/B Sports Bra,* £30.00, movingcomfort.eu.

12. Make resistance exercises fun with this cheerful *Supaflex X-band Exercise Band,* £6.99, physicalcompany.co.uk.

13. The mapped climate control in this Tee targets your high-sweat areas – keeping you dry in all the right places! *C-map Active T-Turquoise Tarn,* £39, stridersedge.com.

GET MORE FROM YOUR WORKOUTS

See best results from your sessions with these easy tips

1 LEAVE STRETCHING UNTIL LATER

A pre-workout stretch may be second nature but the latest sports science research suggests static stretch poses could actually be detrimental to your fitness. Static stretching can shock cold muscles, risking injury and depleting muscle strength by up to 30 per cent, say experts. Limber up with light cardio and some dynamic moves (see page 15) to raise your heart rate and flush your muscles with oxygen. Save those static poses until your cool-down!

2 TURN UP THE MUSIC

There's nothing like uplifting music to boost your exercise endurance. Not only is it a distraction, it's also a rousing performance tool. Studies show some exercisers who listen to music put in up to 10 per cent more effort without realising it. For the best results, choose tracks with a beat that matches the pace of your workout. Optimal exercise music is between 135 and 190 beats per minute. If you need some help compiling the perfect soundtrack, visit www.audiofuel.co.uk.

3 CHECK YOUR POSTURE

It sounds simple, but it's surprising how many people don't give posture a thought when they exercise. Perfect posture – shoulders open and relaxed, spine straight and core muscles engaged – ensures you target the right muscles and work to your capacity. It's also an absolute must for preventing injury, particularly lower back strain.

Before any dynamic movement, remember the posture drill: move your shoulder blades out and down to broaden your upper body and tighten the muscles around your midriff. Never hold your breath during a lifting exercise – breathe in deeply as you prepare for the move and breathe out through pursed lips as you lift.

4 BUDDY UP

Exercising with a friend or trainer has many motivational benefits. For starters, you're less likely to skip sessions if there's someone waiting for you at the gym or park. You can check each other's form and get competitive in cardio sessions to maximise intensity. There is strength in numbers – buddying up is also a good safety tip if you decide to train outdoors.

5 DO MORE IN LESS TIME

Make every minute of your workout count. Research shows that people who spend a long time in the gym often clock up 'dead miles'. Thirty minutes of exercise working at 80 per cent of capacity (eight on the Scale of Perceived Exertion, see page 19) is as good as an hour at 60 per cent. A study published in *The Journal of Applied Physiology* found people who reduced the length of their workouts by 25 per cent could still improve their fitness, provided they boosted the intensity.

6 KEEP YOUR BODY GUESSING

You won't get fitter by doing the same thing day in, day out. Aside from being dull, your body gets used to the routine and stops developing new muscle. To make progress, change your workout every few weeks. Increase the weight of your dumbbells, perform more reps in a set time or make subtle changes to your exercises – for instance, add a resistance band. For cardio, cross-train in a variety of activities, rather than sticking to one exercise type, and up the intensity of your workouts using the Scale of Perceived Exertion. Mix up swimming strokes or do a trail run rather than pounding pavements.

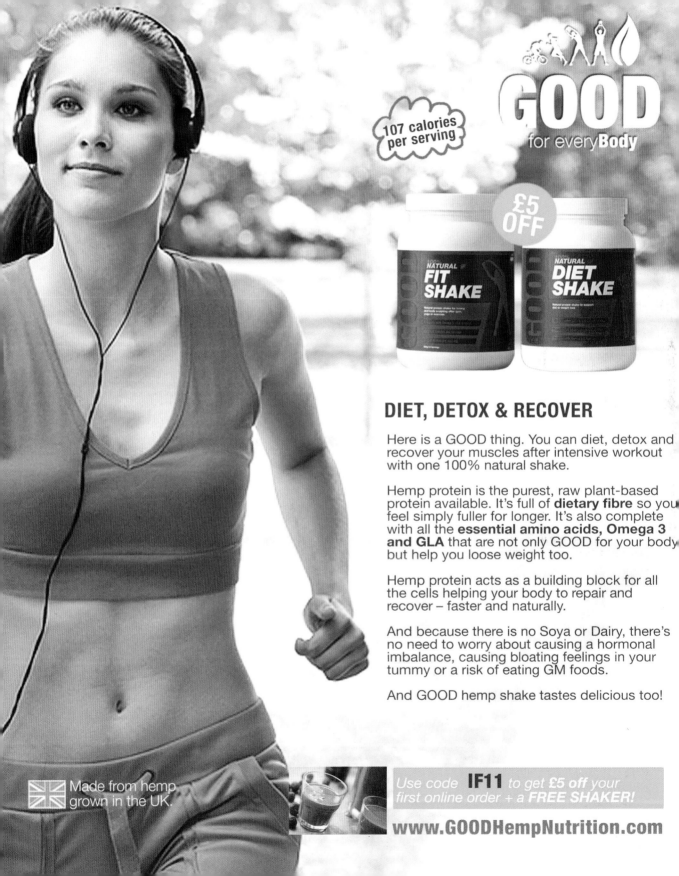

107 calories per serving

£5 OFF

GOOD
for every**Body**

DIET, DETOX & RECOVER

Here is a GOOD thing. You can diet, detox and recover your muscles after intensive workout with one 100% natural shake.

Hemp protein is the purest, raw plant-based protein available. It's full of **dietary fibre** so you feel simply fuller for longer. It's also complete with all the **essential amino acids, Omega 3 and GLA** that are not only GOOD for your body but help you loose weight too.

Hemp protein acts as a building block for all the cells helping your body to repair and recover – faster and naturally.

And because there is no Soya or Dairy, there's no need to worry about causing a hormonal imbalance, causing bloating feelings in your tummy or a risk of eating GM foods.

And GOOD hemp shake tastes delicious too!

Made from hemp grown in the UK.

Use code **IF11** to get **£5 off** your first online order + a **FREE SHAKER!**

www.GOODHempNutrition.com

Training myths
BUSTED!

Time to put misleading exercise folklore to bed.

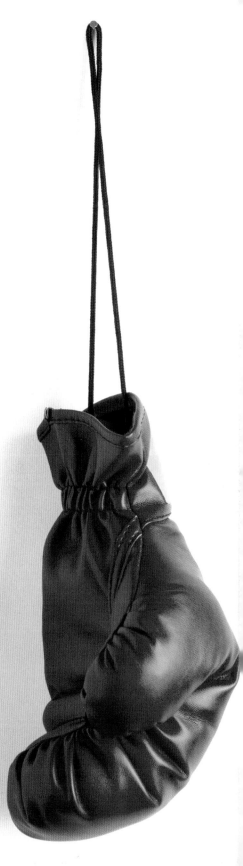

1. 'Resistance training will make me bulky'

Don't worry. You're absolutely not going to turn into an Incredible Hulk-a-like by doing a weights workout once a week. On the contrary, strength training is a flab-fighting tool – lean muscle burns calories even when the body is resting.

2. 'I haven't lost weight – my programme isn't working!'

Yes it is – the more muscle you have, the heavier you'll be. So forget about jumping on the scales. The best way to monitor your progress is to go by the fit of your clothes. Use a tape measure to keep tabs on your vital statistics or ask for a body composition test at your gym. Your fat-to-muscle ratio is much more important than your weight. You may not be shedding pounds but you'll be losing all-important inches.

3. 'Crunches will give me a flat stomach and triceps dips will banish my bingo wings…'

If only things were that easy! You can't spot reduce one area of the body – which is why the exercises in this book are designed to engage various muscle groups simultaneously. The only way you'll achieve a lean, lithe silhouette is through an all-over body plan and sensible eating habits to help you lose fat and increase your lean muscle.

4. 'I need to exercise every day'

The old adage 'all work and no play' applies here – it is possible to exercise too much. Not only does over-exerting yourself cause exhaustion and turn you into a bit of a bore, but it can also compromise your immune system and heighten your risk of injury. Your body needs time to replenish and recover, and build that all-important new muscle tissue.

5. 'Cardio is better than weights for fat loss and definition'

One is neither better than the other. The very best way to strip away fat, sculpt, tone and lift your body is through a combination of cardio and strength training. Building lean muscle through strength training helps boost your metabolism and burn calories even when you're resting.

6. 'Machines are better than free weights'

Absolutely not. Machines have their merits – if you're a beginner you may find them less daunting, for instance. However, for versatility and challenge, you can't beat free weights (such as dumbbells or kettlebells). Not only are they thrifty and adaptable, crucially, they kickstart your stabilising muscles, balance and coordination. Start light and build up slowly to prevent injury.

7. 'No pain, no gain'

While it's true that you have to push yourself to fire up your fitness, pain definitely isn't desirable and may indicate an injury. You should progressively 'overload' your body, training just outside your comfort zone but not beyond it. Mild discomfort is fine; agony is not.

MAMMOTH

Proven to enhance sleep

Dr. Jason Ellis

You will sleep better
We can prove it

The Mammoth Mattress Range brings you unparalleled comfort and support using the latest innovations in sleep science.

Independent research by Northumbria University's Sleep Research Centre proved that Mammoth Mattresses provide a better quality and more enjoyable night sleep so you wake up feeling refreshed and ready to take on the day's challenges.

The Mammoth Mattress Range is available nationwide through selected retailers.

Visit www.mammothmattress.com to find your local retailer

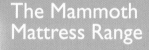

The Mammoth Mattress Range

A breakthrough in sleep science

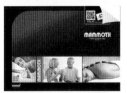

Go to mammothmattress.com and request your free information pack and take your first step to the best night's sleep you can get.

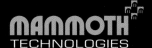

MAMMOTH
TECHNOLOGIES

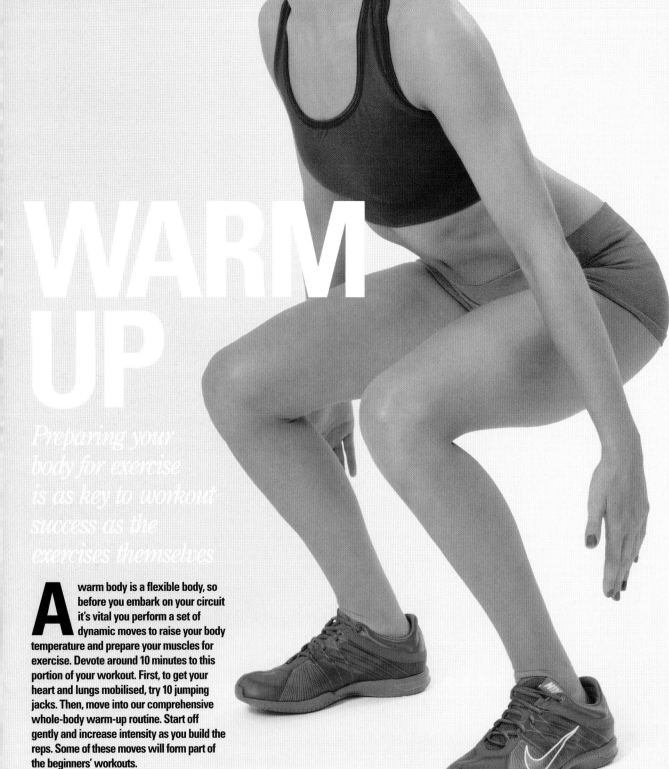

WARM UP

Preparing your body for exercise is as key to workout success as the exercises themselves

A warm body is a flexible body, so before you embark on your circuit it's vital you perform a set of dynamic moves to raise your body temperature and prepare your muscles for exercise. Devote around 10 minutes to this portion of your workout. First, to get your heart and lungs mobilised, try 10 jumping jacks. Then, move into our comprehensive whole-body warm-up routine. Start off gently and increase intensity as you build the reps. Some of these moves will form part of the beginners' workouts.

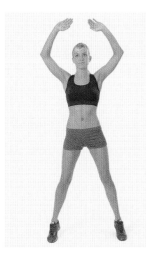

JUMPING JACKS

Stand with your feet together, hands by your sides and knees slightly bent. Engage your abdominals and keep your eyes looking forwards. Simultaneously jump and separate your legs, swinging your arms upward and touching them overhead.

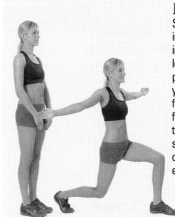

LUNGE TO FLYE

Stand with your arms down in front of your body, palms in. Step forward with your left leg, bend both knees and perform a lunge, spreading your arms wide, palms forwards. Keep your eyes front and back straight throughout. Step back into a standing position and repeat on the right. Do 10 reps on each side.

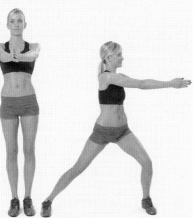

SIDE LUNGE WITH TWIST

Stand with arms extended at shoulder height and hands clasped. Step into a side lunge with your left leg, and rotate your torso and arms in the same direction. Keep your eyes on your hands. Return to the start and repeat on the other side. Do 10 reps on each side.

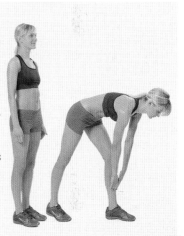

ALTERNATING SPLIT DEADLIFT

Stand with your arms by your sides, then step forward with your left leg. Keeping a slight bend in both knees, lean over your leading leg and extend your arms down, making sure to lean from your hips and keep your spine straight. Return to the start and repeat on the right side. Do 20 reps, 10 on each side.

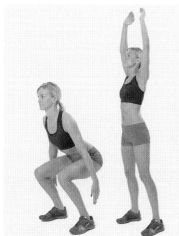

SQUAT TO REACH

With your feet slightly more than shoulder-width apart, arms down by your sides and back straight, perform a simple squat. Hold, then power up through your feet, straighten your legs and raise your arms above your head, keeping your eyes forward. Return to the starting position and repeat 10 times.

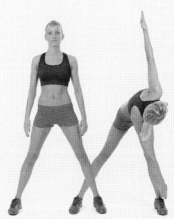

CROSSOVER TOUCH AND REACH

Stand with your feet wider than shoulder width, hands by your sides. Bend forward from the hips and twist your torso while reaching for your right foot with your left hand. Meanwhile, extend your right arm up and look at your hand. Return to the centre and repeat on the other side. Do 10 reps on each side.

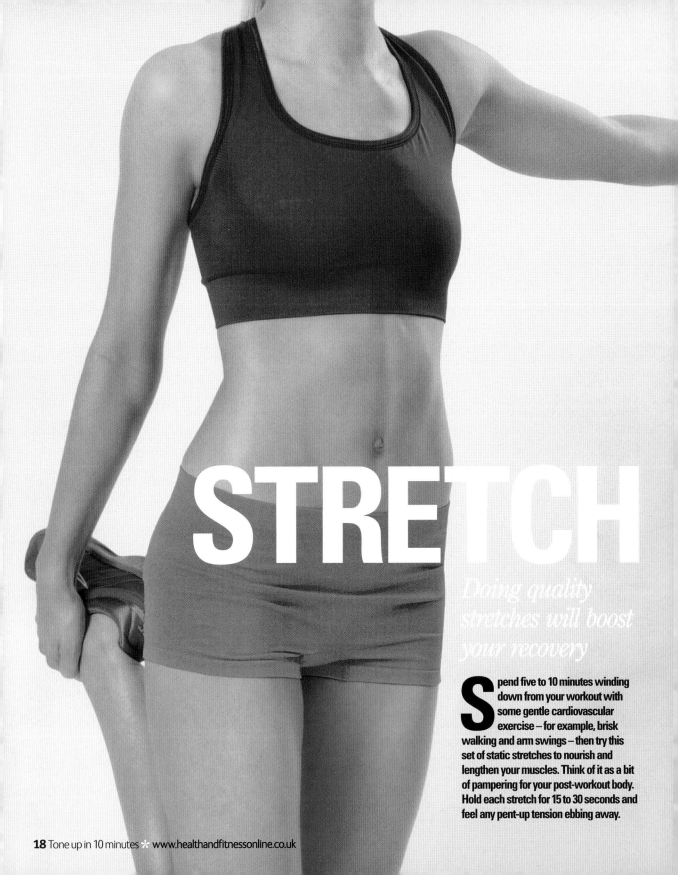

STRETCH

Doing quality stretches will boost your recovery

Spend five to 10 minutes winding down from your workout with some gentle cardiovascular exercise – for example, brisk walking and arm swings – then try this set of static stretches to nourish and lengthen your muscles. Think of it as a bit of pampering for your post-workout body. Hold each stretch for 15 to 30 seconds and feel any pent-up tension ebbing away.

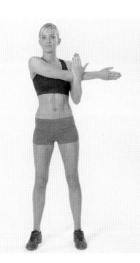

SHOULDERS

Stand tall, feet slightly wider than shoulder width, knees slightly bent. Place your right arm across the front of your chest, parallel to the ground. Ease your right arm closer to your chest with your left forearm. Repeat on the other side.

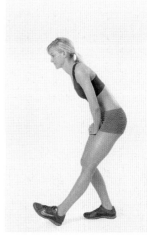

HAMSTRINGS

Stand with your left leg just in front of the right. Bend your right knee and tilt your hips as you rest your weight on your upper right thigh. Your front leg should be straight, toes pointing up. Repeat on the other leg.

TRICEPS

Stand with your feet slightly wider than shoulder width. Slide your right hand up, over your head and down the middle of your spine. Push gently on your right elbow with your left hand. Repeat on the other side.

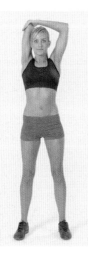

QUADRICEPS

Keeping your back straight, hold on to your right foot and lift it towards your bottom. Extend your left arm out at shoulder height. Keep your knees in line throughout the stretch. Repeat on the left side.

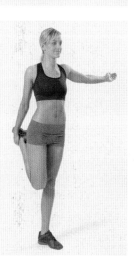

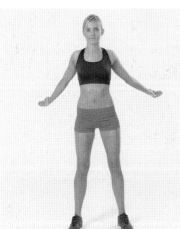

CHEST

Stand and extend your arms out and back as far as is comfortable, with your palms facing away from you. Hold, then repeat.

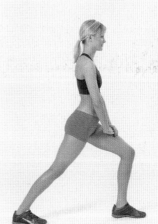

CALVES

Stand tall, then step forward on your left leg, keeping both feet flat on the floor and your right leg straight. Gently bend your left knee and rest your hands on your upper left thigh. Hold, then repeat on the other leg.

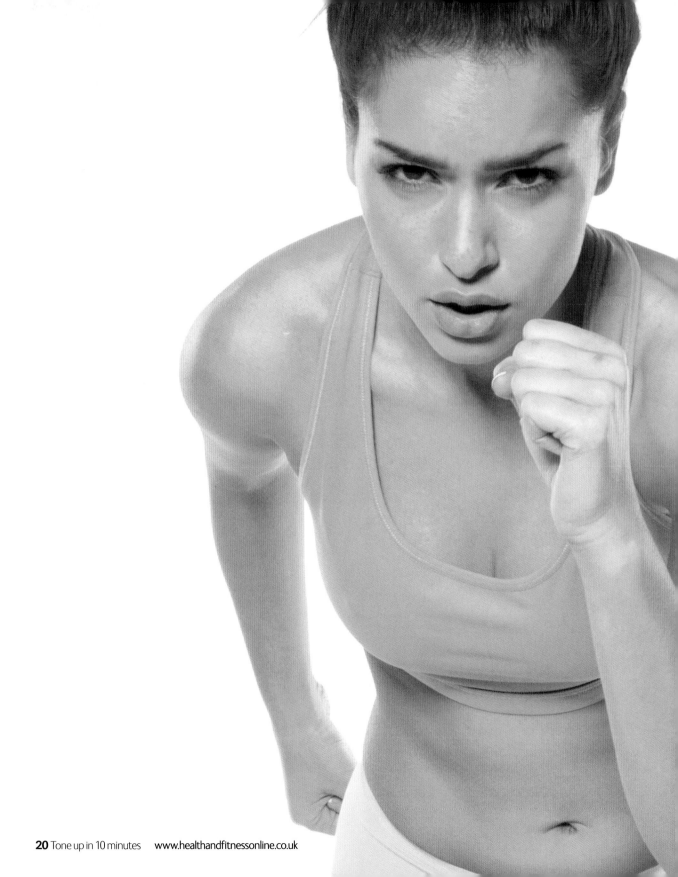

CARDIO

Want to scorch fat and sculpt muscle? For years, scientists believed super-long aerobic workouts offered the best fat-loss rewards. News flash! Slow and steady sessions are relics of the past. Short and speedy is the way to go. Let's take cardio to the next level.

1 **Go hard, not long.** Forget pounding the pavements for hours. A landmark study printed in *The Journal of Applied Physiology* has sparked a craze for speedy interval sessions. And quite rightly so, as data shows 30-second intervals produce the same aerobic benefits as 90 minutes of endurance work.

2 **Hone your exercise habits.** You don't have to be a gym bunny to get your daily exercise dose. Evidence now suggests that injecting small bouts of physical activity into your day – such as taking the stairs, walking to the shops or doing the chores – boasts just as many benefits as a structured workout.

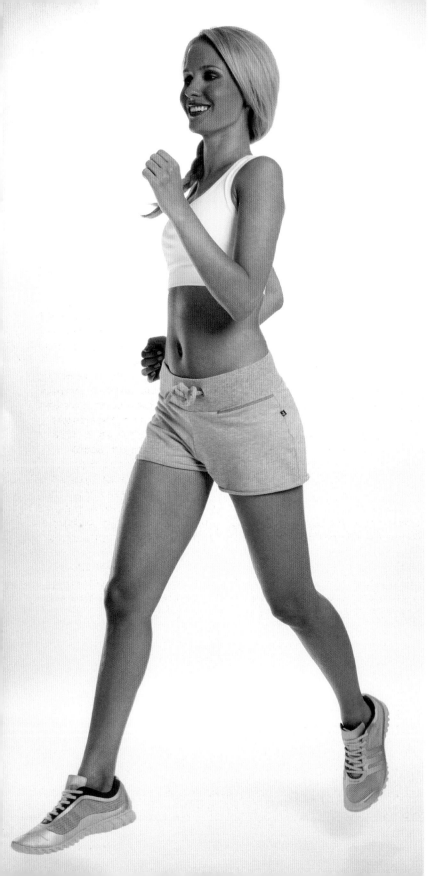

GO GO CARDIO!

No shape-up plan is complete without aerobic activity…

While resistance and strength work ensure sleek bodywork or toned muscles, the smooth running of your heart and lungs – which together make up your body's engine – depend on cardio exercise. At the right level of intensity, cardio kicks your circulatory system into action, fiendishly burns calories, releases mood-enhancing endorphins and brings colour to your cheeks. The two work in perfect harmony.

YOUR CARDIO CHOICES…

WALKING

Cardio doesn't get more accessible, but the benefits are ultra-sophisticated. It uses the same muscles as running – with considerably less impact on the joints – strengthening thighs, hips and bum, and burning upwards of 150 calories an hour, depending on your effort level.

SWIMMING

Did you know the resistance created by water means 30 minutes of activity in the pool is equivalent to 45 minutes of the same activity on land? Although it places no load on the body, swimming is a whole-body workout – it engages all the main muscle groups, burns more than 200 calories in 30 minutes – even at a steady pace – and is a great stress-reliever.

RUNNING

Running can't be beaten for weight loss – even at a moderate pace. A 12-minute-mile pace will burn approximately 250 calories in just half an hour. As well as toning up your major muscle groups, it's great for building bone density (repeated impact with the ground builds skeletal strength) and increasing lung capacity.

CYCLING

Cycling is one of the most popular recreational activities in the UK. Stress-busting, accessible, low-impact and a great calorie-burner (around 600 calories in one hour at a moderate pace), cycling tones up the thighs, calves and bum. Add hills for extra benefits.

DANCING

Since the dawn of *Strictly*, dancing has undergone a massive image overhaul. As well as burning up to 300 calories per hour, toning up your waist, hips and legs,

research shows that memorising complex dance routines sharpens your cognitive function, too. From salsa to street, Bhangra to belly, there's a type to suit every personality.

AEROBICS

Available in a myriad of forms – Bodypump, Boxercise, Hulaerobics and Zumba included – aerobics classes are a great way to haul yourself out of an exercise rut. In addition to cardio work, they combine flexibility, core strength and resistance training in a heady mix, and the mood-lifting class environment keeps your motivation primed. Mix and match your cardio pursuits to add even more spice to your weekly workout regime.

TEAM SPORTS

Cast aside your memories of PE. Team activities such as netball, hockey, softball, volleyball and football have all the cardio benefits you could wish for – with added pizzazz. Studies show that the collective bonding experience of team sports is fabulous for emotional wellbeing, while tactical play tests your cognitive agility.

Top tips

Bust boredom during your longer workouts by trying these ideas:

1 Think about a goal you have. It doesn't have to be realistic – it could be anything from dancing with George Clooney to fitting into your jeans. Just let your mind wander and enjoy the boost!

2 Get into a rhythm. Use music or just the rhythm of your feet hitting the pavement. Focus on it, connect to it and let it carry you along.

3 When you're on a cardio machine, imagine you're in the great outdoors and visualise a journey that takes you over hills, along smooth, flat roads, over bumpy moguls and alongside flowing rivers.

4 If you're training outside, visualise your route as a map in your mind. Keep focusing on the next road, gate, lamppost or corner, until you reach your finishing line.

5 Focus on your core and posture. Keep checking them as you work up a sweat.

YOUR WEEKLY PLAN

Here's an easy way to fit your toning and cardio sessions into your week. For the 10-minute workouts, pick a different part of your body to train each time.

Mon	Tues	Wed	Thurs	Fri	Sat	Sun
10-MINUTE WORKOUT	CARDIO SESSION	10-MINUTE WORKOUT	REST	CARDIO SESSION	10-MINUTE WORKOUT	REST

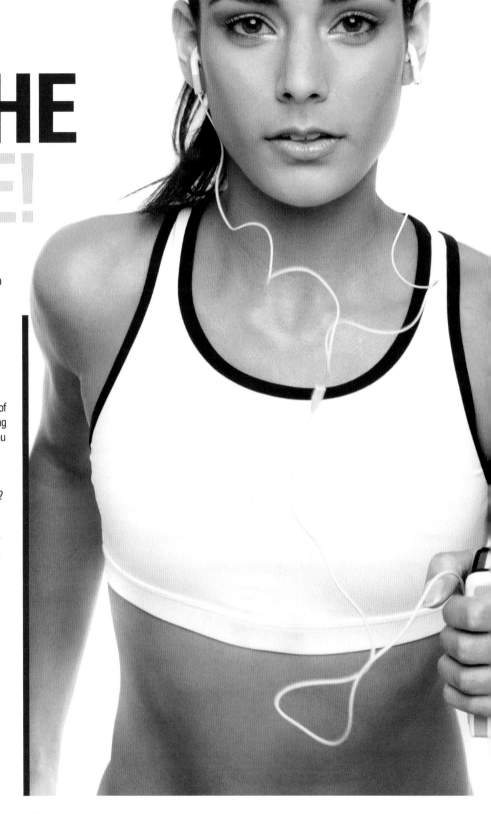

UP THE PACE!

Slow and steady doesn't win the race, so crank up the cardio

Want to spend less time sweating over every cardio workout and more time living your life? Good news. Long, slow aerobic exercise – distance runs, two-hour swims and the like – is no longer king of the calorie killers. Instead, an increasing amount of research is showing that you can compress all your exercise into a few minutes and reap the same rewards. Exercise less; get better results – sounds far-fetched, doesn't it? Surprisingly, it's not. High-intensity interval training (better known by the acronym HIIT to gym junkies) is a new way to work out – and it has taken the global fitness scene by storm.

What is HIIT?

There's good reason why HIIT exercise is the go-to workout. The HIIT format – brief intervals of near-maximal-intensity exercise teamed with easy activity for recovery – is proven to burn off more calories per minute than a longer workout at a steady pace. So how is that achieved? At slower speeds, your body's primary fuel source is fat, while at higher intensities it draws on carbohydrate circulating in the blood and muscles. For this reason, exercisers have long believed that slow-speed workouts equal more fat loss.

The truth is, the more calories you burn, the more weight you lose, regardless of what type of fuel the energy comes from. And HIIT workouts burn a lot of calories, mainly because high-intensity training recruits fast-twitch muscle fibres. These fibres produce powerful bursts of energy and need plenty of fuel to do it. The result? The body uses up more energy and burns lots of calories.

So, less is more – and not just for your fitness, but for your health as well. Indeed, scientists at the University of Montreal found that HIIT improves brain oxygenation, boosting mental capacity. And that's not all – exercisers also showed increased insulin sensitivity, which is important for keeping your blood sugar levels stable and reducing your risk of developing Type 2 diabetes.

What does it do?

Not convinced? HIIT is backed up by a lot of science. Leading the HIIT movement is a study from McMaster University in Canada. The Canadian researchers split exercisers into two groups – one group did 90-120 minutes of easy cycling three times a week; the other group completed two to three minutes of intense interval cycling, again, three times a week. After a fortnight, results showed that both sets of participants had increased their body's mitochondria stores (the cells' energy factories that boost oxygen consumption). To be clear, six minutes of weekly intervals turned out to be as great for aerobic fitness as 300 minutes of exercising at a moderate pace.

HIIT also makes your heart stronger. Another study, printed in the *American Journal of Physiology*, showed that high-intensity exercise, at 90-95 per cent of maximal oxygen consumption (known as VO_2 max to those in science circles), increased left ventricle heart mass by an impressive 12 per cent. This near-maximal training method also improved cardiac contractility by an even bigger 13 per cent. The net result is a sturdier ticker and greater cardiovascular health.

And there's more, HIIT training also primes aerobic performance. Activities such as cycling, swimming and running rely on getting oxygen to exercising muscles. Greater oxygen consumption means you swim, cycle or run faster, and research suggests that HIIT is better than endurance training for improving it. Such research, printed in the *Journal of Physiology*, measured VO_2 max responses among participants following either an eight-week HIIT or week endurance plan. The HIIT exercisers increased their VO_2 max by a whopping 15 per cent, while the endurance workout produced only a nine per cent boost. Scientists conclude that HIIT training ups aerobic fitness, but over fewer sessions and a shorter period of time than endurance training.

The catch, of course, is that HIIT workouts hurt, as training bouts need to be intense – anything above seven on the rate of perceived exertion (RPE), where one is nothing at all and 10 is all-out effort – to produce the best results. But don't be put off this cardio option as it's a great way to hone a hotter body. Experts at the University of Guelph discovered that women doing two weeks of HIIT exercise increased their bodies' ability to burn fat while they moved. Hurrah!

Q How hard do I have to exercise?

A Pioneering HIIT researchers describe a bout of HIIT work as 'all-out effort' or 'well out of your comfort zone'. What's your comfort zone? Think of it as the slightly-breathy sensation you get on a steady-paced bike ride or the feeling of running an easy pace during a long jog. For HIIT training, start at that pace, then crank the intensity up a notch for 10 seconds to a couple of minutes. Simple.

Q Do I need to be super fit to do a HIIT workout?

A HIIT is not for the fainthearted. If you haven't been exercising regularly, consult a doctor before beginning a HIIT programme. That said, if you're a beginner exerciser, you can still benefit from HIIT training. Begin with two to three weekly HIIT sessions of moderate intensity and build it over two months. This will give your body time to adjust to the increase in intensity.

Q Am I wasting my time doing long cardio?

A HIIT training is a great way to improve your cardiovascular fitness, but slow and steady sessions still have a place in your fitness schedule. Longer workouts are a fantastic way to boost VO_2 max, heart health and muscular strength, plus they're easy on your body and are sustainable day after day. Use slow-speed workouts to boost your base fitness levels, and support your HIIT training plan by doing two to three HIIT workouts and one to two moderate sessions per week.

TAKE A HIIT

Ready to give HIIT a go? Try one of our favourite
HIIT workouts to benefit from the fat-frying method

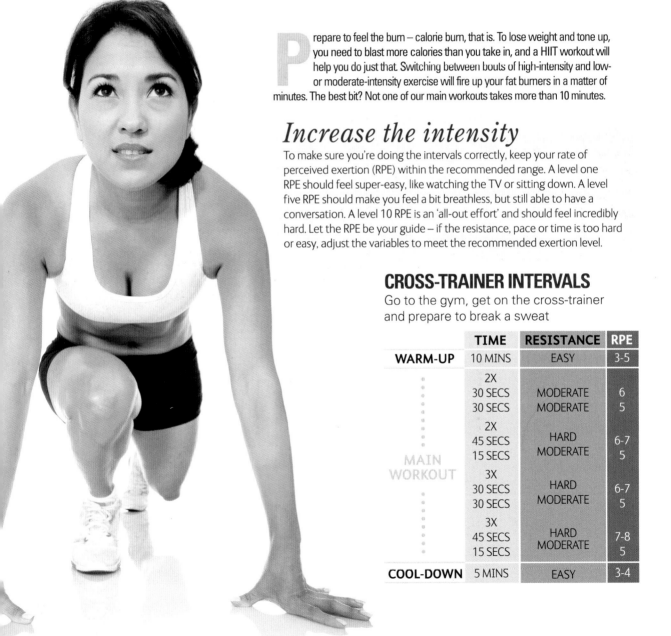

repare to feel the burn – calorie burn, that is. To lose weight and tone up,
you need to blast more calories than you take in, and a HIIT workout will
help you do just that. Switching between bouts of high-intensity and low-
or moderate-intensity exercise will fire up your fat burners in a matter of
minutes. The best bit? Not one of our main workouts takes more than 10 minutes.

Increase the intensity

To make sure you're doing the intervals correctly, keep your rate of
perceived exertion (RPE) within the recommended range. A level one
RPE should feel super-easy, like watching the TV or sitting down. A level
five RPE should make you feel a bit breathless, but still able to have a
conversation. A level 10 RPE is an 'all-out effort' and should feel incredibly
hard. Let the RPE be your guide – if the resistance, pace or time is too hard
or easy, adjust the variables to meet the recommended exertion level.

CROSS-TRAINER INTERVALS

Go to the gym, get on the cross-trainer
and prepare to break a sweat

	TIME	RESISTANCE	RPE
WARM-UP	10 MINS	EASY	3-5
	2X 30 SECS 30 SECS	MODERATE MODERATE	6 5
	2X 45 SECS 15 SECS	HARD MODERATE	6-7 5
MAIN WORKOUT	3X 30 SECS 30 SECS	HARD MODERATE	6-7 5
	3X 45 SECS 15 SECS	HARD MODERATE	7-8 5
COOL-DOWN	5 MINS	EASY	3-4

CYCLING HARDY HILLS

Cycle gently to a steep hill and repeatedly
power up it, then pedal slowly back home

	TIME	EFFORT	RPE
WARM-UP	6 MINS	EASY FLAT	3-4
MAIN WORKOUT	2X 2 MINS 1 MIN	HILL SPRINT EASY DOWN HILL	7-8 5
	1X 3 MINS 1 MIN	HILL SPRINT EASY DOWN HILL	7-8 5
COOL-DOWN	6 MINS	FLAT ROAD	3-4

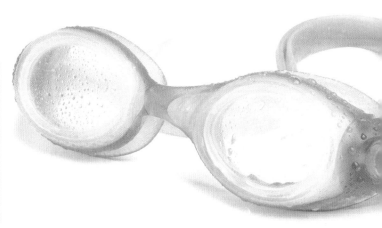

RUNNING SUPER SPRINTS

On a flat road, track or treadmill, run as fast as
you can between the active jog recoveries

	TIME	PACE	RPE
WARM-UP	10 MINS	WALK/JOG	3-4
MAIN WORKOUT	5X 40 SECS 20 SECS	SPRINT JOG	7-8 4-5
	1 MIN	WALK/JOG	4
	2X 1 MIN 1 MIN	SPRINT JOG	7-8 4-5
COOL-DOWN	5 MINS	WALK/JOG	3-5

SWIMMING POOL POWER

Watch the clock and try to beat your sprint time
in the second, same-distance sprint

	PACE	DISTANCE	RPE
WARM-UP	EASY (any stroke)	400 METRES	3-4
MAIN WORKOUT	2X FRONT CRAWL SPRINT EASY (any stroke)	12.5M 12.5M	7-8
	2X FRONT CRAWL SPRINT EASY (any stroke)	25M 25M	7-8
	2X FRONT CRAWL SPRINT EASY (any stroke)	50M 50M	7-8
COOL-DOWN	GENTLE KICKING	200	3-4

ROWING MACHINE MISSION

Row the target distance in the given time,
then try to beat your time on the next round

	TIME	DISTANCE	RPE
WARM-UP	3 MINS	ANY	3-4
MAIN WORKOUT	3 MINS 2 MINS 3 MINS	700 METRES ANY 700 METRES	7-8 3-4 7-8
COOL-DOWN	5 MINS	ANY	3-4

HIIT training is one of the best methods for losing weight and
improving fitness, but that doesn't mean it's going to be easy.
During the high-intensity interval periods, it's important to exercise
as hard as you can – this means no talking, lots of sweating and
plenty of heavy breathing – and try to do it with proper form. The
active rest is there to help you regain a little energy for the next
interval, in which you should be able to exercise just as hard.
REMEMBER, YOU'RE STRONGER THAN YOU THINK!

LET'S GET
PHYSICAL!

Get ready to supercharge your fitness
without stepping foot in the gym

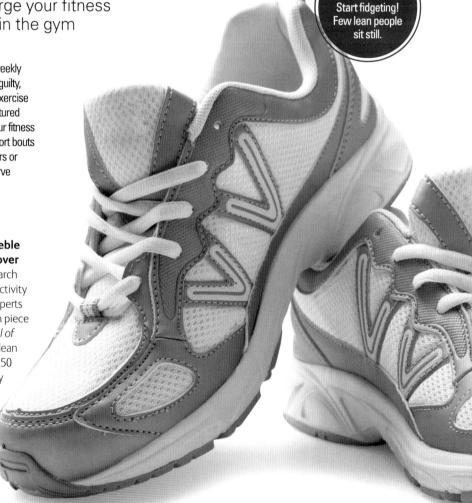

Quick tip!
Start fidgeting!
Few lean people
sit still.

Do you struggle to fit in your weekly training sessions? Don't feel guilty, as you may be doing more exercise than you think. While a structured workout plan is a great way to meet your fitness goals, current wisdom suggests that short bouts of daily activity – such as taking the stairs or washing the car – will crush fat and carve lean muscle, too.

The benefits

While this may sound like a feeble excuse for choosing the telly over a gym session, a plethora of research shows that Non-Exercise Physical Activity – or NEPA, as it's been coined by experts – is impressively effective. One such piece of research, published in the *Journal of Internal Medicine*, discovered that lean participants burned an average of 350 additional calories per day simply by doing more non-exercise activity, such as standing and walking, than their heavier counterparts. To put that in perspective, many people would blast a similar amount of energy on a three-mile jog. As study leader

Dr Levine explains, 'You can expend calories in one of two ways. One is to go to the gym and the other is through the activities of daily living.'

Of course, it's not just calorie expenditure you should be concerned about, as an increasing amount of research is showing that a lack of activity in daily life increases the risk of heart disease, diabetes and other health woes. Data published in the *American Journal of Epidemiology*, for example, discovered that people sitting for fewer than six hours a day lived longer than their sedentary comrades. More recently, experts at the University of Leicester added to this morbid news by discovering that excessive amounts of sitting increases the risk of Type 2 diabetes.

So, why has sitting got such a bad reputation? According to the experts, it's because long periods of inactivity halt the muscle activity that triggers processes related to the breakdown of fats and sugars in the body. Laziness is bad for your health – sounds logical, doesn't it?

Well, gym fanatics can suffer the negative effects of inactivity, too. Research shows that being fit won't necessarily help matters – a structured workout such as gym session or lunchtime run is not the antidote to excessive bouts of sitting.

Instead, scientists claim the answer is to take short and frequent breaks from being sedentary – walk your dog, get up to talk to colleagues or stand occasionally. As an added bonus, evidence suggests this will also reduce metabolic syndrome (a group of risk factors – high blood pressure, high blood sugar, unhealthy cholesterol levels and abdominal fat – that contribute to heart disease risk), thanks to positive changes in the levels of lipoprotein lipase. Sounds simple – right?

How to do it

So should you scrap your gym sessions completely? No, planned workouts will still go a long way to improving your health and wellbeing, as well as boosting specific elements of your fitness such as stamina or power. But non-exercise activity is great for bolstering general fitness, too, and the foundations of NEPA are certainly not new activities. In fact, before technology and industry, most people enjoyed a greater level of non-exercise fitness. It's only in recent years we've chosen to sit down to work, after all.

With this in mind, to up your amount of NEPA, simply aim to be more active in day-to-day life. This increase in activity may include walking to the shops, doing the gardening or cleaning the dishes – they are all examples of non-exercise physical activity. NEPA pioneer Dr Levine says that all of the things we do in the course of the day, whether dancing, going to work, shovelling snow, playing the guitar or walking, count as NEPA. It's simple, so give it a go.

Find your fix

Want to up your daily activity to burn more calories? Here are a few examples of NEPA to try.

1 DO THE HOUSEWORK
Yes, those necessary chores do count as exercise! While cleaning the house may not be the most exciting way to get a fitness fix, consider the upside – you'll burn hoards of calories and then relax in a clean and tidy home afterwards. According to experts, washing the floor or cleaning the car blasts more than 150 calories in just 30 minutes.

2 TIDY THE GARDEN
You can blitz some serious fat during a marathon gardening session. Statistics show you can use up to 200 calories per half hour of gardening, plus going from standing-to-squatting is great for muscle tone! Choose traditional gardening methods to work your body harder, such as feeding the plants with a watering can rather than using a hose.

3 WALK TO WORK
Walking is a great way to boost your leg strength and up cardiovascular fitness. If you live too far away from the office, park your car a few miles away from work and walk the rest of the distance. As a good rule of thumb, you'll torch 100 calories per mile.

4 TAKE MORE BREAKS
According to data, the average adult spends 90 per cent of their leisure time sitting down, and further research shows that reducing sitting time by 90 minutes daily would decrease your risk of Type 2 diabetes. Cut your sedentary time by getting up to talk to colleagues, making more tea at work and going for regular strolls.

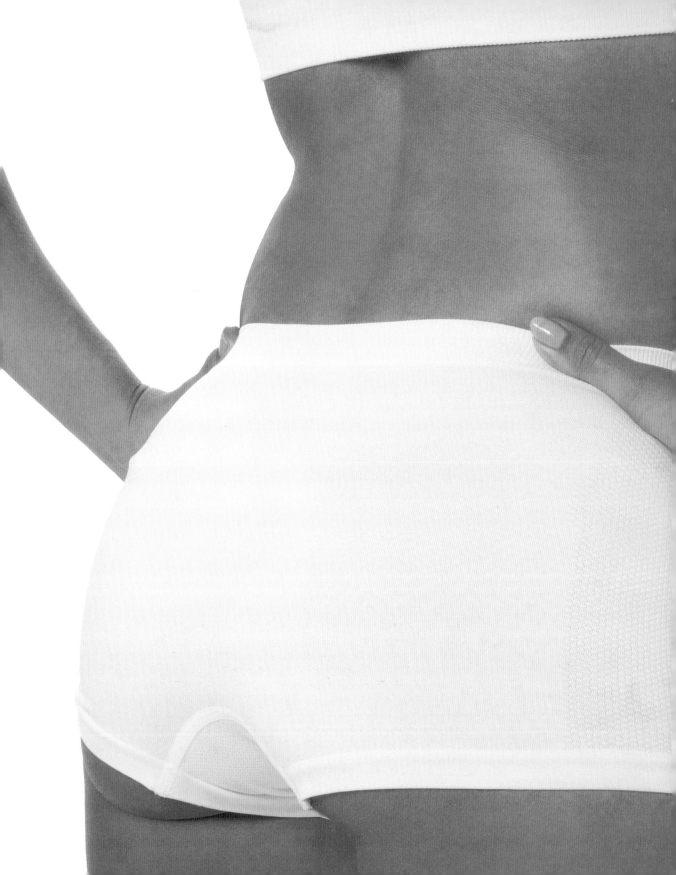

BUM

A pert, peachy bum is top of many a fitness wish list. Although you can't alter its natural shape, there's plenty you can do to shed fat and reveal a more defined, sculpted derrière. This set of gold-standard exercises challenges your gluteal muscle group, to lift and tone your bum.

SIX WAYS TO A PEACHY BOTTOM

1. Take the stairs and walk uphill. You won't firm up your bottom unless you're walking against resistance.

2. Beware 'chair bottom'. Don't sit down when you don't need to. Did you know one in five adults spend over 30 hours a week marooned on their sofas?

3. Tone your skin by dry-brushing. Using a natural bristle, brush your skin before your bath or shower – and don't neglect your bum. Brush in an upward direction from your calves towards your heart.

4. Imagine you have a £20 note between your bum cheeks. Gently keep hold of it by maintaining some 'tone' in your buttocks, but don't over-clench.

5. Think about your posture. If you let your tummy sag out and pelvis tip forward, your gluteals (bottom muscles) are 'on stretch' and aren't working. Keep your pelvis in neutral, slightly tipped back, tummy engaged.

6. Take up kickboxing. Kicks to the back, front and side target your bottom from all directions. You'll burn fat too.

EXERCISE ONE

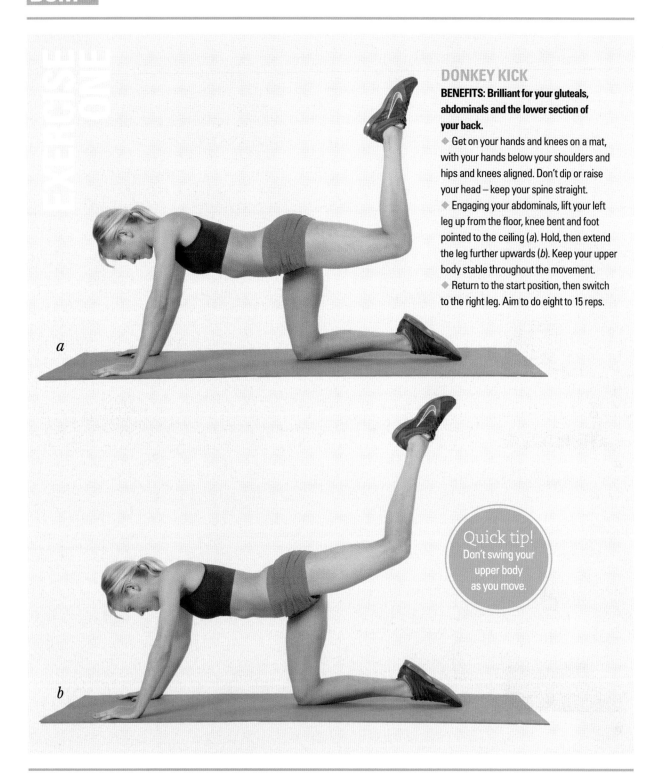

a

b

DONKEY KICK

BENEFITS: Brilliant for your gluteals, abdominals and the lower section of your back.

◆ Get on your hands and knees on a mat, with your hands below your shoulders and hips and knees aligned. Don't dip or raise your head – keep your spine straight.

◆ Engaging your abdominals, lift your left leg up from the floor, knee bent and foot pointed to the ceiling (*a*). Hold, then extend the leg further upwards (*b*). Keep your upper body stable throughout the movement.

◆ Return to the start position, then switch to the right leg. Aim to do eight to 15 reps.

Quick tip!
Don't swing your
upper body
as you move.

LYING LATERAL LEG KICK

BENEFITS: Great for your outer thighs and quadriceps, as well as your abdominals.

◆ Lie on your right side, propping your head up on your right elbow. Your feet should be flexed so you're able to see your toes.

◆ Using your left hand to stabilise you, engage your core and move your top leg backwards (*a*). Keep your hips stable throughout – don't swing your body. Keep your head still and focus straight ahead.

◆ Move your leg in front of you to complete one rep (*b*). Aim to do between eight and 15 reps.

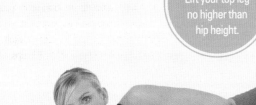

Quick tip!
Lift your top leg
no higher than
hip height.

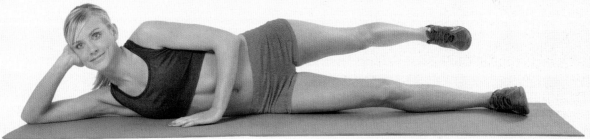

a

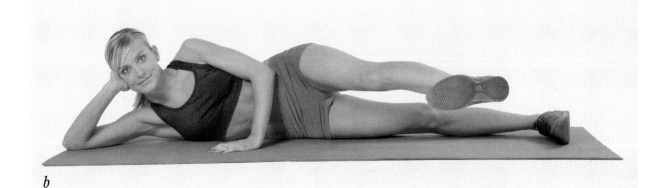

b

EXERCISE THREE

CLOCK LUNGES

BENEFITS: Works your lower body in all three planes of movement to sculpt your gluteals, hamstrings, quadriceps and inner and outer thighs.

◆ Lunge forward at 12 o'clock with your right foot until your right knee is bent at 90° (*a*). Return to a standing position.

◆ Continue lunging with your right leg at two o'clock (*b*), three o'clock (*c*), five o'clock (*d*) and six o'clock (*e*).

◆ Now switch to lunging with your left leg, starting at six o'clock (stepping backwards) and working round the clock – seven o'clock, nine o'clock, 10 o'clock and two o'clock – until you are back at the start.

◆ One complete rep means doing 10 lunges in total. Do one to two reps.

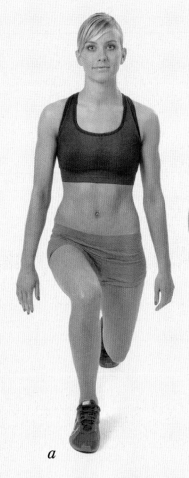

a

Quick tip!
Maintain an upright posture throughout and keep your stomach muscles engaged.

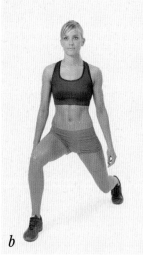

b

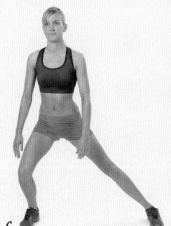

c

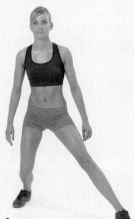

d

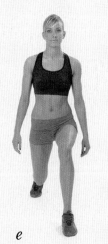

e

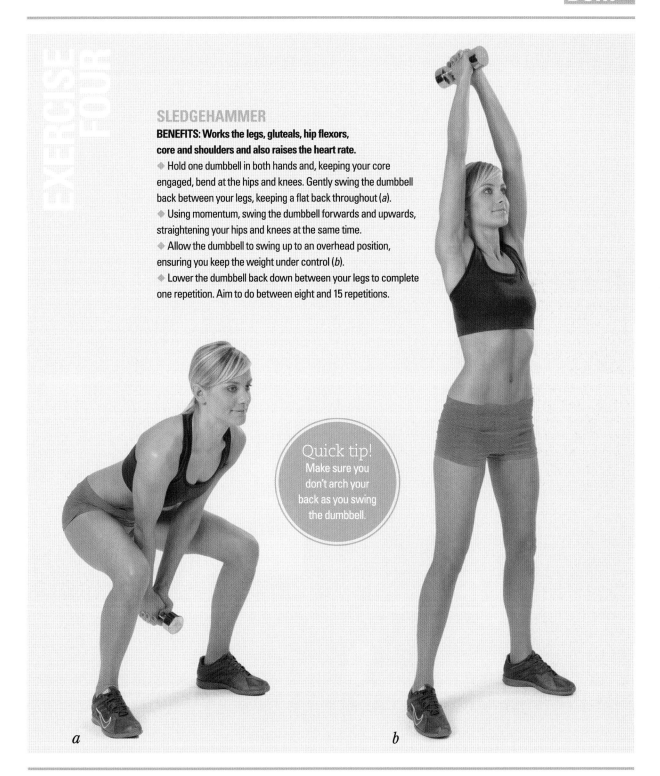

EXERCISE FOUR

SLEDGEHAMMER

BENEFITS: Works the legs, gluteals, hip flexors, core and shoulders and also raises the heart rate.

◆ Hold one dumbbell in both hands and, keeping your core engaged, bend at the hips and knees. Gently swing the dumbbell back between your legs, keeping a flat back throughout (*a*).

◆ Using momentum, swing the dumbbell forwards and upwards, straightening your hips and knees at the same time.

◆ Allow the dumbbell to swing up to an overhead position, ensuring you keep the weight under control (*b*).

◆ Lower the dumbbell back down between your legs to complete one repetition. Aim to do between eight and 15 repetitions.

Quick tip!
Make sure you don't arch your back as you swing the dumbbell.

a

b

EXERCISE FIVE

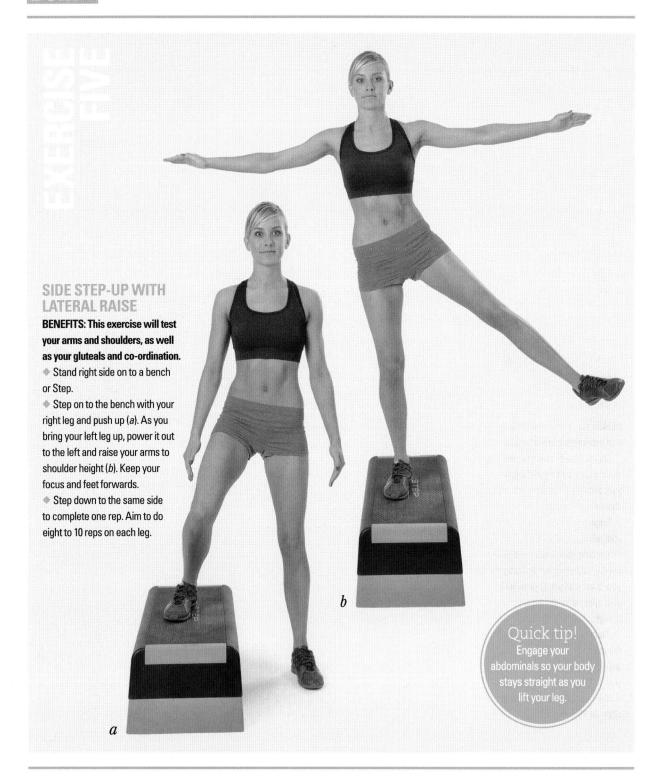

SIDE STEP-UP WITH LATERAL RAISE

BENEFITS: This exercise will test your arms and shoulders, as well as your gluteals and co-ordination.

◆ Stand right side on to a bench or Step.

◆ Step on to the bench with your right leg and push up (*a*). As you bring your left leg up, power it out to the left and raise your arms to shoulder height (*b*). Keep your focus and feet forwards.

◆ Step down to the same side to complete one rep. Aim to do eight to 10 reps on each leg.

a

b

Quick tip!
Engage your abdominals so your body stays straight as you lift your leg.

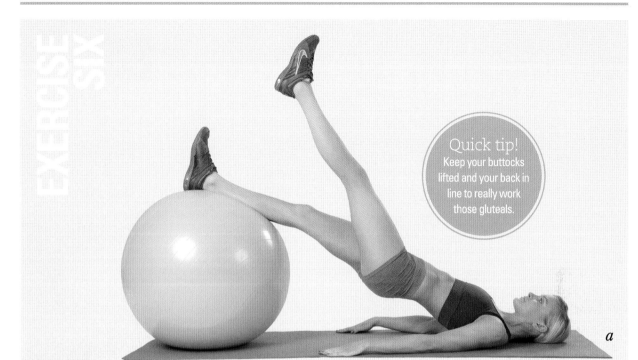

EXERCISE SIX

Quick tip!
Keep your buttocks
lifted and your back in
line to really work
those gluteals.

a

GYM BALL SINGLE LEG CURL

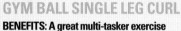

**BENEFITS: A great multi-tasker exercise
that works your lower body and core.**

◆ Lie on a cushioned mat, with your calves
resting on top of a gym ball, feet together and
your arms by your sides. Your neck and shoulders
should be relaxed.

◆ Engaging your abs, raise your hips and lift
your left leg away from the ball (*a*).

◆ Keeping your left leg and hips stable,
bend your right knee and drag the ball towards
your bum with your right heel (*b*). Keep
your spine lifted from the floor and
straight throughout.

◆ Pause for a moment at the top of
the move, then straighten your right
leg again by pushing the ball. Return
your left leg to the ball, and repeat
on the opposite side. Aim to do
eight to 15 reps.

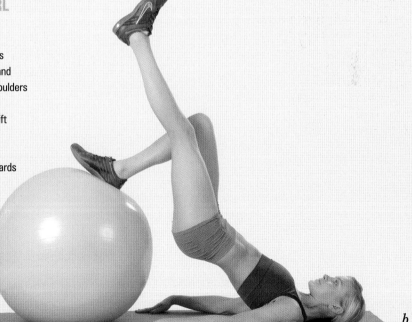

b

EXERCISE SEVEN

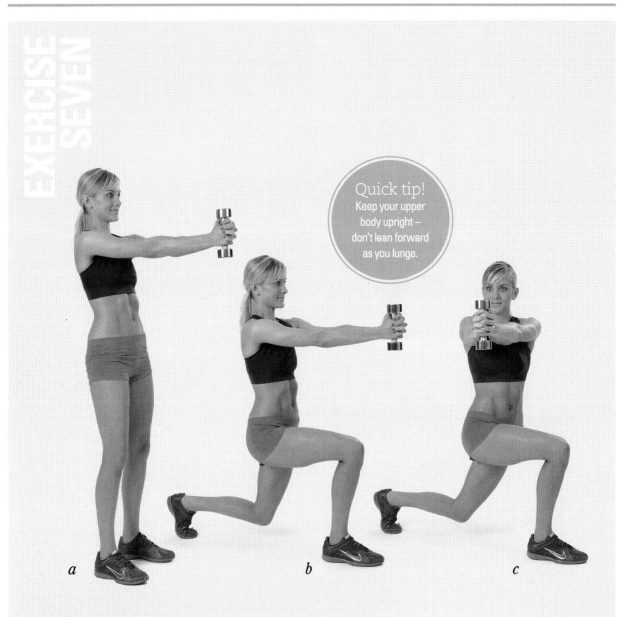

Quick tip!
Keep your upper
body upright —
don't lean forward
as you lunge.

a

b

c

DUMBBELL LUNGE WITH TWIST

BENEFITS: This exercise targets the hamstrings, legs, gluteals and sides of the body, as well as building power and co-ordination.

◆ Stand in a neutral position, grasping a dumbbell with two hands at shoulder height (*a*).

◆ Take a dynamic step forward with your right foot, lunging down (*b*). Then, keeping the dumbbell at shoulder height, twist to your right — your focus should move with your torso (*c*).

◆ Return to the starting position. Aim to do eight to 15 reps.

EXERCISE EIGHT

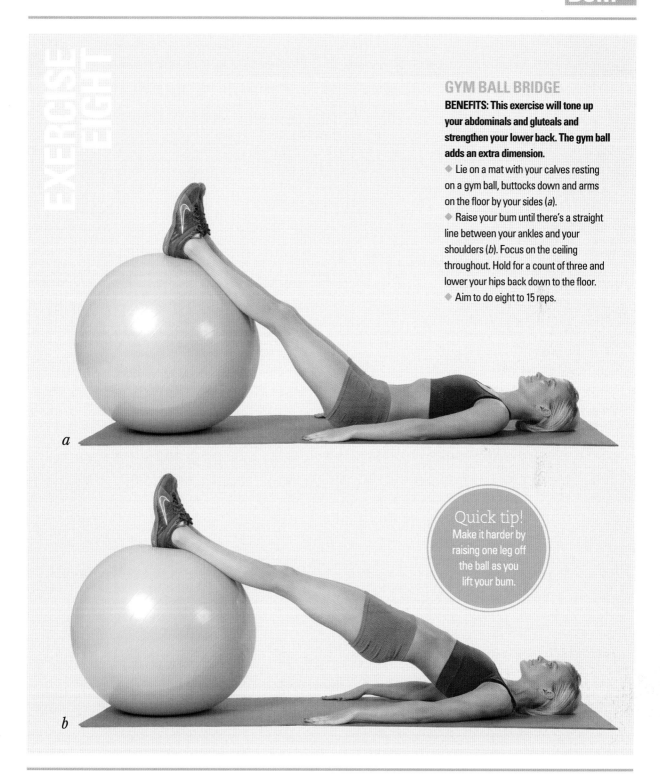

GYM BALL BRIDGE

BENEFITS: This exercise will tone up your abdominals and gluteals and strengthen your lower back. The gym ball adds an extra dimension.

◆ Lie on a mat with your calves resting on a gym ball, buttocks down and arms on the floor by your sides (*a*).

◆ Raise your bum until there's a straight line between your ankles and your shoulders (*b*). Focus on the ceiling throughout. Hold for a count of three and lower your hips back down to the floor.

◆ Aim to do eight to 15 reps.

a

Quick tip!
Make it harder by raising one leg off the ball as you lift your bum.

b

10-MINUTE BUM WORKOUT
BEGINNER

Gym novices can ease themselves in with this no-kit circuit.

WHAT TO DO... After warming up your muscles, perform this circuit twice, resting for one minute between each circuit. Finish with some stretching.

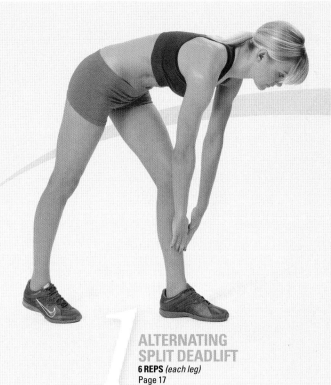

1 ALTERNATING SPLIT DEADLIFT
6 REPS *(each leg)*
Page 17

EXERCISES	REPS/DURATION	PAGE
1. ALTERNATING SPLIT DEADLIFT	**6 REPS** *(each leg)*	17
REST	30 SECONDS	
2. CLOCK LUNGE (CLOCKWISE)	**1 REP** *(10 lunges)*	34
REST	30 SECONDS	
3. DONKEY KICK	**6 REPS** *(each leg)*	32
REST	30 SECONDS	
4. CLOCK LUNGE (ANTI-CLOCKWISE)	**1 REP** *(10 lunges)*	34
REST	30 SECONDS	
5. LYING LATERAL LEG KICK	**6 REPS** *(each leg)*	33
REST	1 MINUTE	

REST 1 MINUTE

5 LYING LATERAL LEG KICK
6 REPS *(each leg)*
Page 33

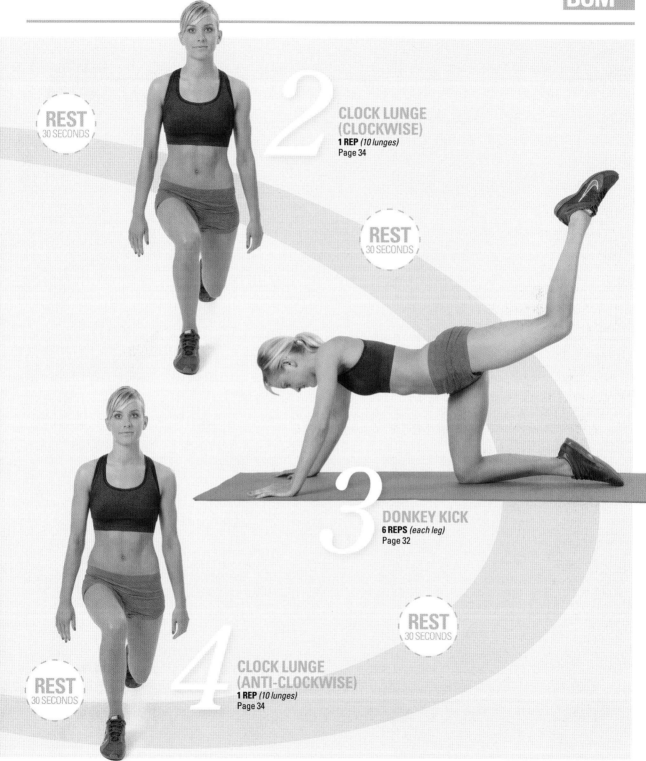

REST
30 SECONDS

2 CLOCK LUNGE
(CLOCKWISE)
1 REP *(10 lunges)*
Page 34

REST
30 SECONDS

3 DONKEY KICK
6 REPS *(each leg)*
Page 32

REST
30 SECONDS

4 CLOCK LUNGE
(ANTI-CLOCKWISE)
1 REP *(10 lunges)*
Page 34

REST
30 SECONDS

10-MINUTE
BUM WORKOUT
INTERMEDIATE

*Move up to the next level
with this intermediate
challenge for your gluteals.*

WHAT TO DO... This workout comprises a
giant set – three exercises combined –
sandwiched between two sets of clock lunges.
You'll do three giant sets in all, resting 30
seconds between each, and the high intensity
will help raise your metabolism and torch fat.

EXERCISES	REPS/DURATION	PAGE
1. CLOCK LUNGE	**2 REPS** *(both directions 20 lunges)*	34
REST	1 MINUTE	
2a. JUMPING JACKS	**30 SECONDS**	17
2b. GYM BALL BRIDGE	**8 REPS** *(hold each for 3 counts)*	39
2c. LYING LATERAL LEG KICK	**6 REPS** *(each leg)*	33
REST	1 MINUTE	
3. CLOCK LUNGE	**2 REPS** *(both directions 20 lunges)*	34

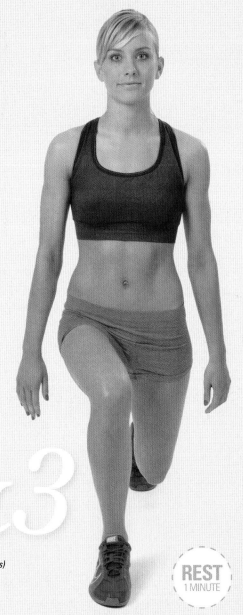

1&3

CLOCK LUNGE
2 REPS *(both directions 20 lunges)*
Page 34

REST
1 MINUTE

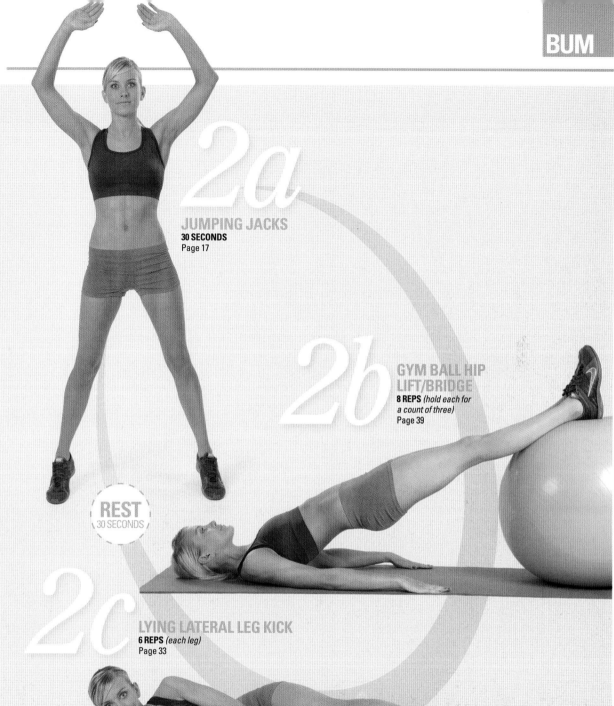

2a
JUMPING JACKS
30 SECONDS
Page 17

2b
GYM BALL HIP LIFT/BRIDGE
8 REPS *(hold each for a count of three)*
Page 39

REST
30 SECONDS

2c
LYING LATERAL LEG KICK
6 REPS *(each leg)*
Page 33

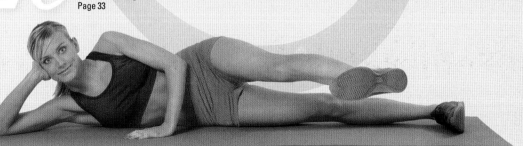

10-MINUTE BUM WORKOUT ADVANCED

Crank up the effort with this expert circuit.

WHAT TO DO… Grab your dumbbells, gym ball and Step or bench for this high-octane circuit. Perform it three times, moving seamlessly from one exercise to the next, resting for one minute after each circuit.

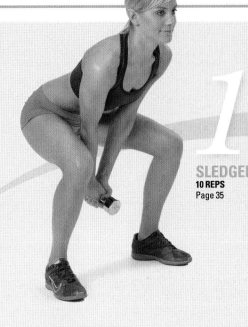

1

SLEDGEHAMMER
10 REPS
Page 35

EXERCISES	REPS/DURATION	PAGE
1. SLEDGEHAMMER	**10 REPS**	35
2. GYM BALL SINGLE LEG CURL	**5 REPS** *(each leg)*	37
3. SIDE STEP-UP WITH LATERAL RAISE	**5 REPS** *(each leg)*	36
4. DONKEY KICK	**5 REPS** *(each leg)*	32
5. DUMBBELL LUNGE WITH TWIST	**10 REPS** *(alternating sides)*	38
REST	1 MINUTE	

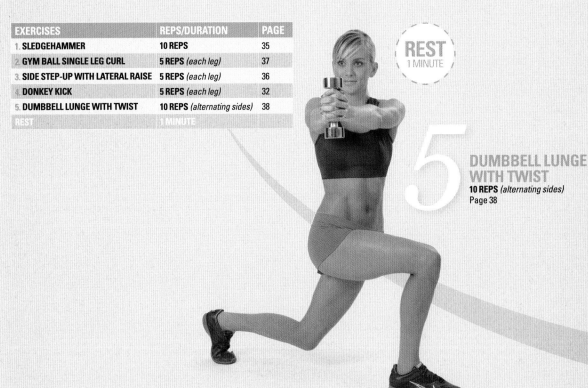

REST
1 MINUTE

5

DUMBBELL LUNGE WITH TWIST
10 REPS *(alternating sides)*
Page 38

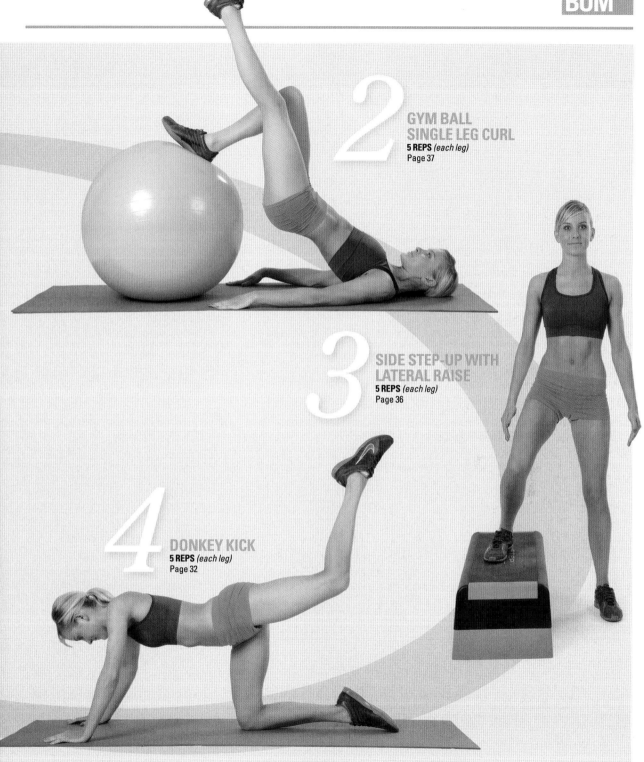

2 GYM BALL SINGLE LEG CURL
5 REPS *(each leg)*
Page 37

3 SIDE STEP-UP WITH LATERAL RAISE
5 REPS *(each leg)*
Page 36

4 DONKEY KICK
5 REPS *(each leg)*
Page 32

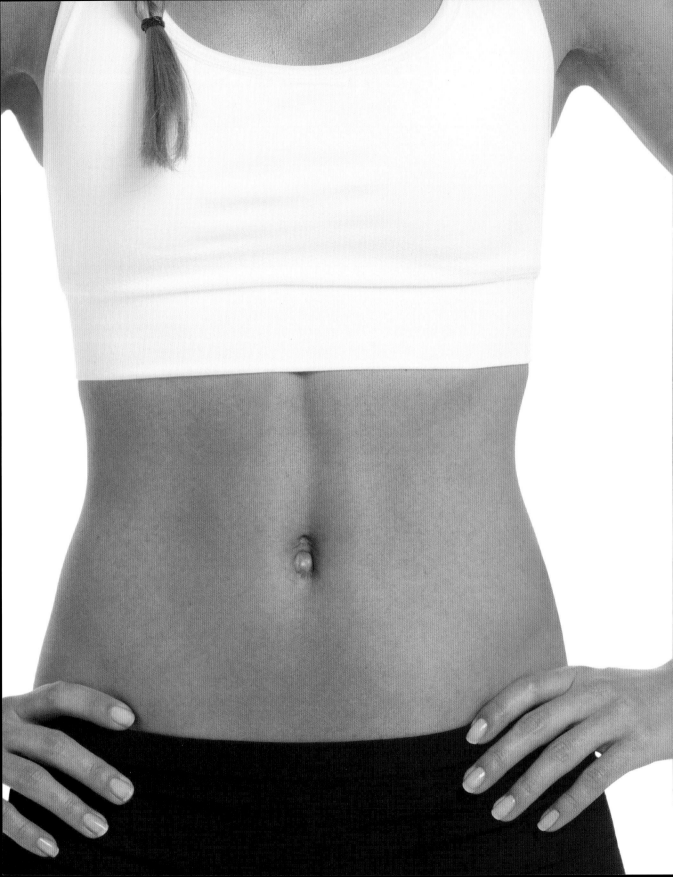

ABS

Bare your midriff with pride. This set of moves will tone not only your 'six-pack' muscles, but also the sides of your waist and the all-important deep core muscles that hold your tummy in.

SIX WAYS TO A FLAT BELLY

1. Engage your core muscles in your daily life. Every time you bend down or reach up for something, switch them on by pulling your belly button towards your spine and keeping your abdominals tight.
2. Stand up when you're doing resistance exercises such as bicep curls and shoulder raises. This forces your core region to work harder to stabilise you.
3. Tie a piece of string around your waist while your abdominals are gently engaged. Leave it there all day and you'll be reminded to draw your tummy in every time you feel your skin pressing against the string.
4. Think about your posture! You can instantly 'lose' inches by drawing in your tummy, opening up your chest and dropping your shoulders and ribcage.
5. A gym ball is a star piece of kit for toning your abs. As well as using one during workouts, use it as an alternative to a chair.
6. Try belly-dancing – it challenges your oblique muscles at the sides of the waist.

EXERCISE ONE

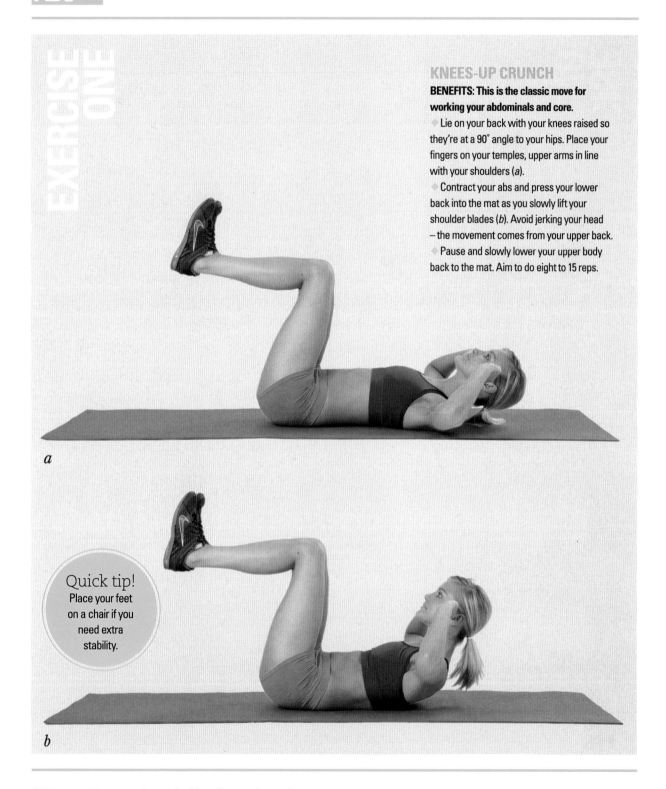

KNEES-UP CRUNCH

BENEFITS: This is the classic move for working your abdominals and core.

◆ Lie on your back with your knees raised so they're at a 90° angle to your hips. Place your fingers on your temples, upper arms in line with your shoulders (*a*).

◆ Contract your abs and press your lower back into the mat as you slowly lift your shoulder blades (*b*). Avoid jerking your head – the movement comes from your upper back.

◆ Pause and slowly lower your upper body back to the mat. Aim to do eight to 15 reps.

a

Quick tip!
Place your feet on a chair if you need extra stability.

b

EXERCISE TWO

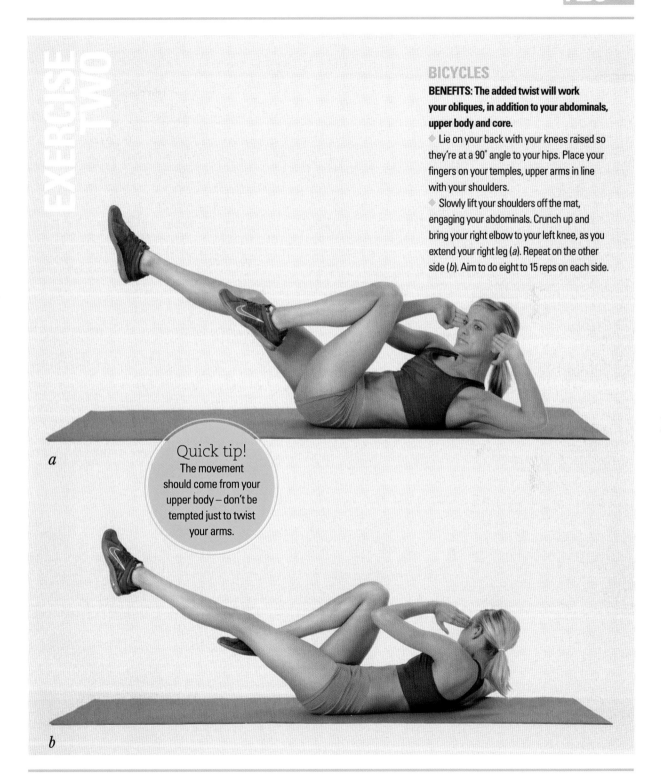

BICYCLES

BENEFITS: The added twist will work your obliques, in addition to your abdominals, upper body and core.

◆ Lie on your back with your knees raised so they're at a 90° angle to your hips. Place your fingers on your temples, upper arms in line with your shoulders.

◆ Slowly lift your shoulders off the mat, engaging your abdominals. Crunch up and bring your right elbow to your left knee, as you extend your right leg (*a*). Repeat on the other side (*b*). Aim to do eight to 15 reps on each side.

a

Quick tip!
The movement should come from your upper body – don't be tempted just to twist your arms.

b

EXERCISE THREE

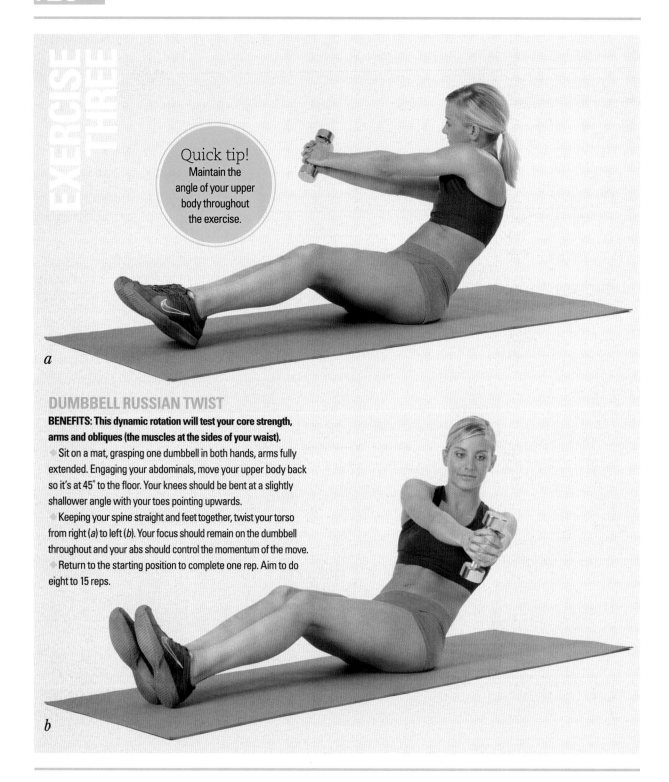

Quick tip!
Maintain the angle of your upper body throughout the exercise.

a

DUMBBELL RUSSIAN TWIST

BENEFITS: This dynamic rotation will test your core strength, arms and obliques (the muscles at the sides of your waist).

◆ Sit on a mat, grasping one dumbbell in both hands, arms fully extended. Engaging your abdominals, move your upper body back so it's at 45° to the floor. Your knees should be bent at a slightly shallower angle with your toes pointing upwards.

◆ Keeping your spine straight and feet together, twist your torso from right (*a*) to left (*b*). Your focus should remain on the dumbbell throughout and your abs should control the momentum of the move.

◆ Return to the starting position to complete one rep. Aim to do eight to 15 reps.

b

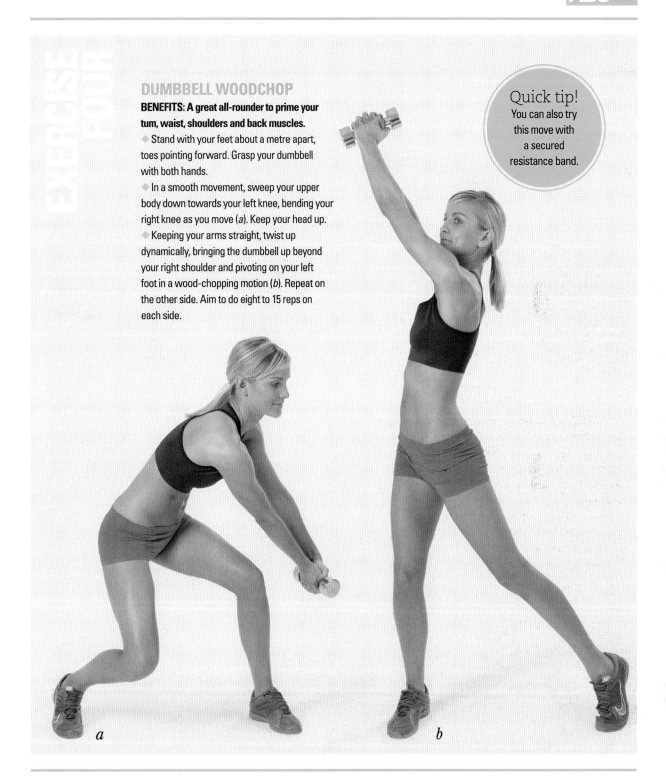

EXERCISE FOUR

DUMBBELL WOODCHOP

BENEFITS: A great all-rounder to prime your tum, waist, shoulders and back muscles.

◆ Stand with your feet about a metre apart, toes pointing forward. Grasp your dumbbell with both hands.

◆ In a smooth movement, sweep your upper body down towards your left knee, bending your right knee as you move (*a*). Keep your head up.

◆ Keeping your arms straight, twist up dynamically, bringing the dumbbell up beyond your right shoulder and pivoting on your left foot in a wood-chopping motion (*b*). Repeat on the other side. Aim to do eight to 15 reps on each side.

Quick tip!
You can also try this move with a secured resistance band.

a

b

EXERCISE FIVE

a

Quick tip!
Keep your feet
planted on
the floor
throughout.

GYM BALL CRUNCH WITH TWIST

BENEFITS: The addition of a gym ball tests your stabilising muscles and allows you to achieve a wider range of movement.

◆ Lie back on a gym ball with your upper body supported. Your feet should be positioned below your hips, your fingers on your temples, upper arms in line with your shoulders (*a*).

◆ Engage your core and slowly lift your upper body from the ball. As you do so, twist your torso to the left (*b*). Keep your neck in line with your spine throughout the movement. Repeat on the other side to complete a rep.

◆ Aim to do eight to 15 reps.

b

EXERCISE SIX

SIDE PLANK

BENEFITS: A plank with added benefits! This move will challenge your core muscles, arms and waist.

◆ Lie on your side with your weight resting on your right elbow, keeping it directly below your shoulder. Place your left foot on top of the right – keep your feet flexed and your toes pointing forward.

◆ Hold your body in a straight line from head to feet, making sure you keep your hips lifted throughout. Aim to hold for 30 seconds to a minute, then repeat on the other side.

Quick tip!
For an extra challenge, lift your upper arm away from your body.

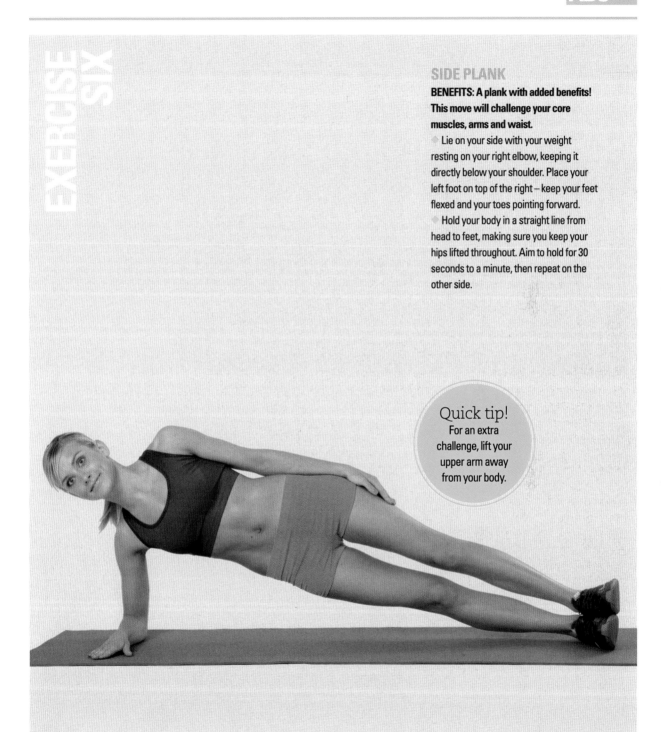

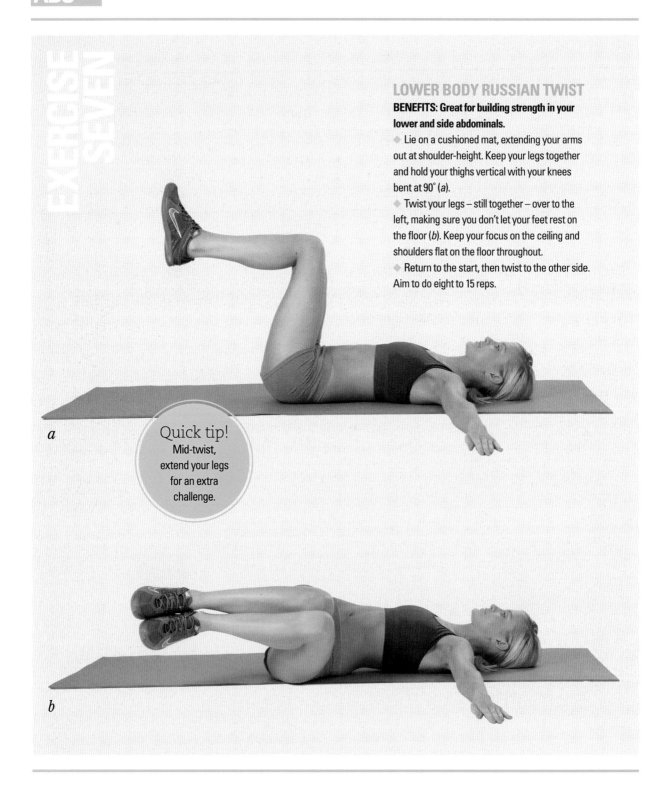

EXERCISE SEVEN

LOWER BODY RUSSIAN TWIST

BENEFITS: Great for building strength in your lower and side abdominals.

◆ Lie on a cushioned mat, extending your arms out at shoulder-height. Keep your legs together and hold your thighs vertical with your knees bent at 90° (*a*).

◆ Twist your legs – still together – over to the left, making sure you don't let your feet rest on the floor (*b*). Keep your focus on the ceiling and shoulders flat on the floor throughout.

◆ Return to the start, then twist to the other side. Aim to do eight to 15 reps.

a

Quick tip!
Mid-twist, extend your legs for an extra challenge.

b

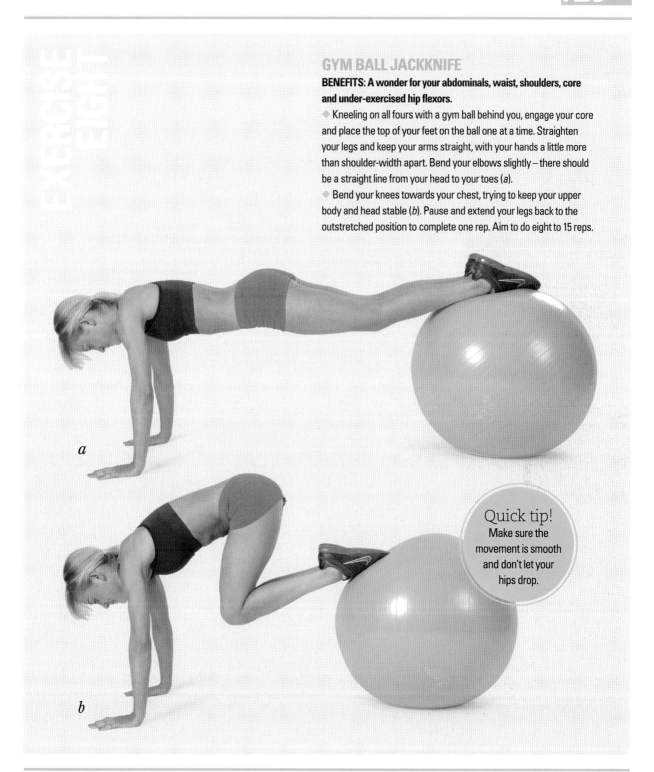

EXERCISE EIGHT

GYM BALL JACKKNIFE

BENEFITS: A wonder for your abdominals, waist, shoulders, core and under-exercised hip flexors.

◆ Kneeling on all fours with a gym ball behind you, engage your core and place the top of your feet on the ball one at a time. Straighten your legs and keep your arms straight, with your hands a little more than shoulder-width apart. Bend your elbows slightly – there should be a straight line from your head to your toes (*a*).

◆ Bend your knees towards your chest, trying to keep your upper body and head stable (*b*). Pause and extend your legs back to the outstretched position to complete one rep. Aim to do eight to 15 reps.

a

b

Quick tip!
Make sure the movement is smooth and don't let your hips drop.

10-MINUTE ABS WORKOUT BEGINNER

A no-equipment circuit for toned abs.

WHAT TO DO... After warming up, move through this circuit twice, resting for 30 seconds in between each exercise and for 30 seconds between circuits. No equipment required, other than a cushioned mat.

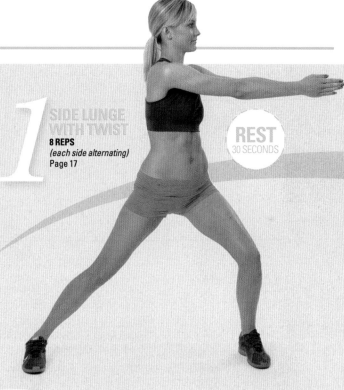

1 SIDE LUNGE WITH TWIST
8 REPS
(each side alternating)
Page 17

REST
30 SECONDS

EXERCISES	REPS/DURATION	PAGE
1. SIDE LUNGE WITH TWIST	**8 REPS** *(each side alternating)*	17
REST	30 SECONDS	
2. KNEES-UP CRUNCH	**8 REPS** *(or as many as you can)*	48
REST	30 SECONDS	
3. CROSSOVER TOUCH AND REACH	**8 REPS** *(each side alternating)*	17
REST	30 SECONDS	
4. SIDE PLANK (RIGHT THEN LEFT)	**30 SECONDS** *(each side)*	53
REST	30 SECONDS	
5. LOWER BODY RUSSIAN TWIST	**5 REPS** *(each side)*	54
REST	30 SECONDS	

REST
30 SECONDS

5 LOWER BODY RUSSIAN TWIST
5 REPS *(each side)*
Page 54

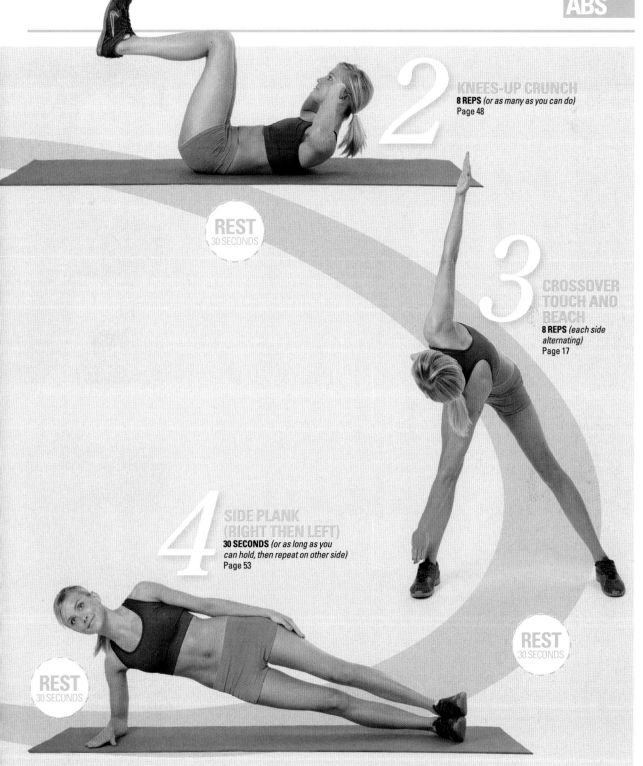

2 KNEES-UP CRUNCH
8 REPS (or as many as you can do)
Page 48

3 CROSSOVER TOUCH AND REACH
8 REPS (each side alternating)
Page 17

4 SIDE PLANK (RIGHT THEN LEFT)
30 SECONDS (or as long as you can hold, then repeat on other side)
Page 53

REST
30 SECONDS

REST
30 SECONDS

REST
30 SECONDS

10-MINUTE ABS WORKOUT INTERMEDIATE

A high-octane intermediate abs circuit.

WHAT TO DO... With dumbbells and mat close by, try this powerful circuit three times over. Don't rest between exercises – you have a one-minute break awaiting you after each circuit.

EXERCISES	DURATION	PAGE
1. JUMPING JACKS	30 SECONDS	17
2. BICYCLES	30 SECONDS	49
3. SQUAT TO REACH	30 SECONDS	17
4. AQUAMAN	30 SECONDS	100
5. DUMBBELL RUSSIAN TWIST	30 SECONDS	50
REST	1 MINUTE	

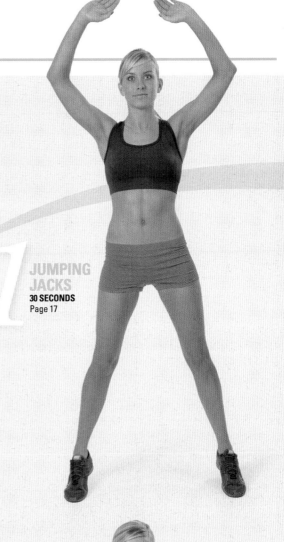

1 JUMPING JACKS
30 SECONDS
Page 17

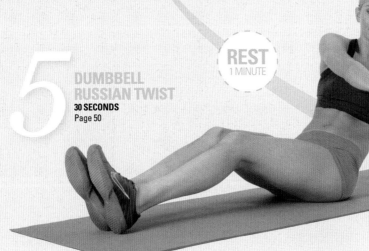

5 DUMBBELL RUSSIAN TWIST
30 SECONDS
Page 50

REST
1 MINUTE

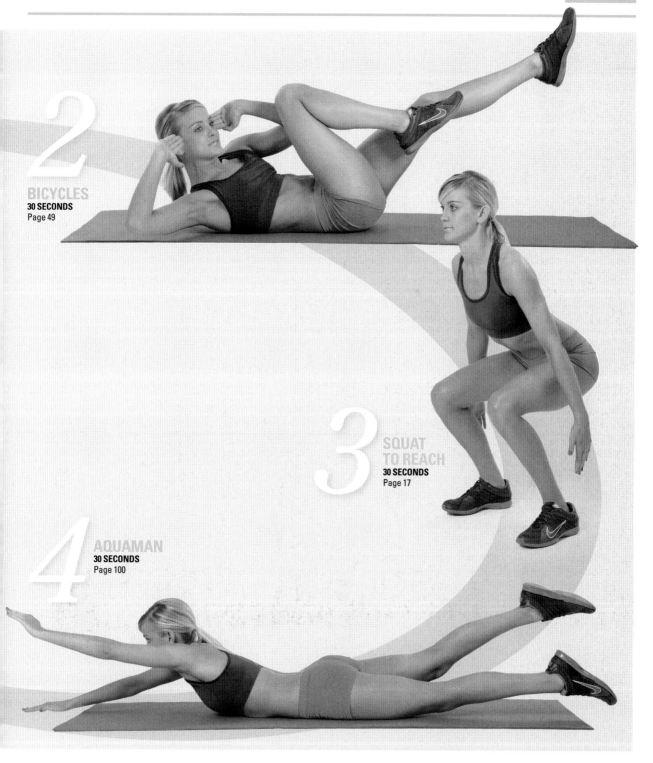

2
BICYCLES
30 SECONDS
Page 49

3
SQUAT TO REACH
30 SECONDS
Page 17

4
AQUAMAN
30 SECONDS
Page 100

10-MINUTE ABS WORKOUT ADVANCED

Give your abdominals an advanced test.

WHAT TO DO... This workout for gym regulars comprises a four-part circuit, performed four times, plus an added side plank challenge. You'll need your dumbbells and gym ball. Perform exercises one to four, then repeat three more times resting for 30 seconds between each circuit. Once you've completed the four circuits, do the two sets of planks.

EXERCISES	REPS/DURATION	PAGE
1. DUMBBELL WOODCHOP (LEFT)	12 REPS	51
2. GYM BALL CRUNCH WITH TWIST	12 REPS *(alternating)*	52
3. DUMBBELL WOODCHOP (RIGHT)	12 REPS	51
4. GYM BALL JACKKNIFE	12 REPS	55
REST	30 SECONDS	
5. SIDE PLANK (LEFT)	1 MINUTE	53
6. SIDE PLANK (RIGHT)	1 MINUTE	53

1

DUMBBELL WOODCHOP (LEFT TO RIGHT)
12 REPS
Page 51

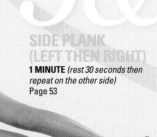

5&6

SIDE PLANK (LEFT THEN RIGHT)
1 MINUTE *(rest 30 seconds then repeat on the other side)*
Page 53

REST
30 SECONDS

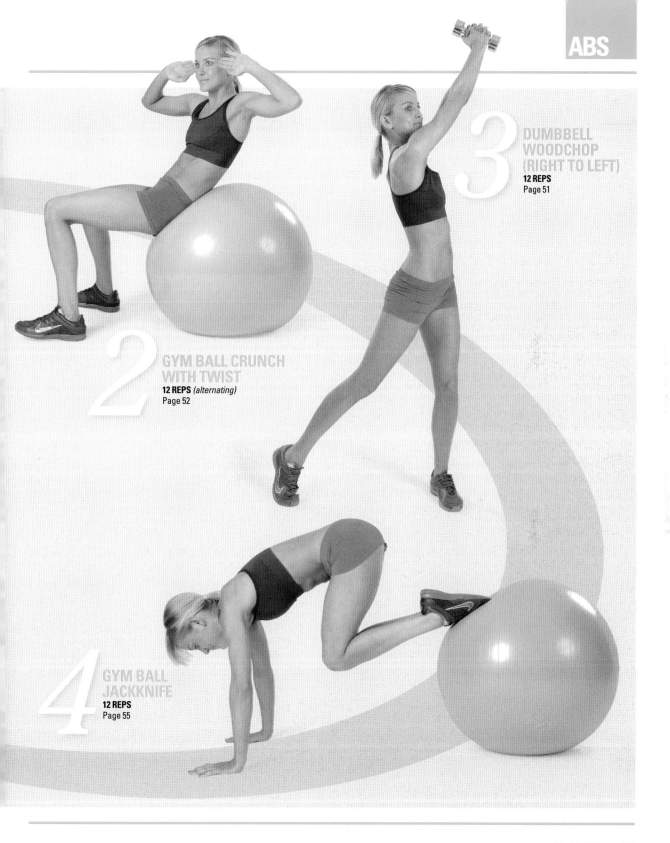

3

DUMBBELL WOODCHOP (RIGHT TO LEFT)
12 REPS
Page 51

2

GYM BALL CRUNCH WITH TWIST
12 REPS *(alternating)*
Page 52

4

GYM BALL JACKKNIFE
12 REPS
Page 55

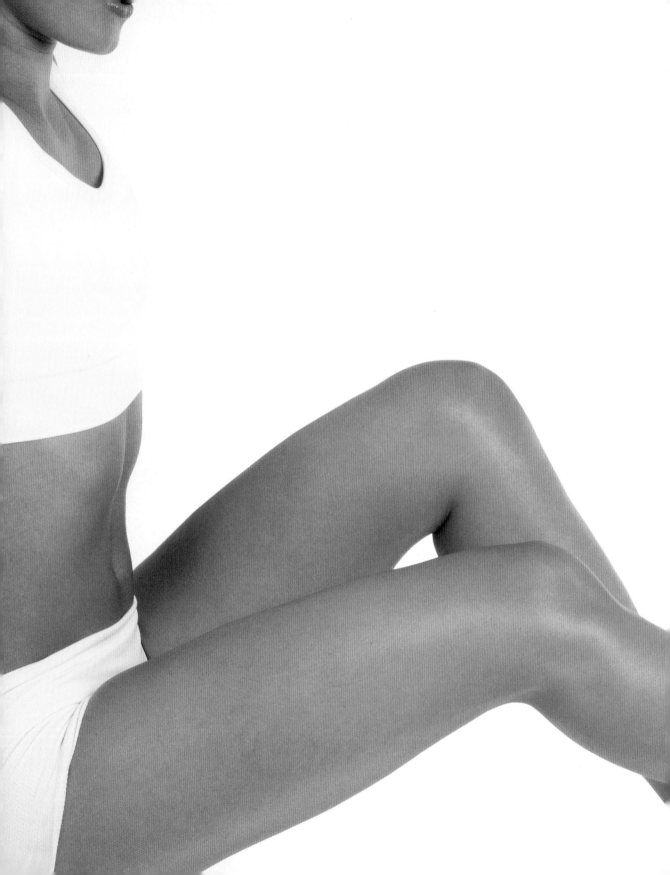

LEGS

If your goal is perfect pins, you've come to the right place. This section is all about getting those toned, lean and shapely legs you've always dreamed of.

SIX WAYS TO HOT LEGS

1. Walking, running and cycling are all fabulous for your legs. Work them into your daily routine by 'active commuting' – eschewing the car, bus or train and getting to work at least partly under your own steam.
2. If you can't get out for a brisk walk or run, try the boxer's cardiovascular exercise of choice: skipping. It's great for your hips and bum as well as your legs.
3. Give a ballet class a try. It's fantastic for elongating and streamlining the lower body, as well as challenging your core.
4. Legs look better when they're bronzed – just remember to exfoliate before you slap on the fake tan.
5. Minimise cellulite by avoiding processed and fatty foods and eating more antioxidant-rich fruit and vegetables and good fats from nuts and oily fish.
6. Tone-while-you-walk footwear helps firm up your legs and tweak your posture.

EXERCISE ONE

LYING LATERAL LEG RAISE

BENEFITS: Great for the sides of your stomach as well as your bum and thighs.

◆ Lie on your right side, with hips stacked and your head propped up by your right hand (*a*).

◆ Keeping your body in a straight line and your toes pointing forward, raise your left leg, making sure you don't roll your pelvis as you move (*b*).

◆ Pause, then lower your leg to complete one rep. Aim to do eight to 15 reps on each side.

a

Quick tip!
Use an ankle weight on your top leg to increase the effort.

b

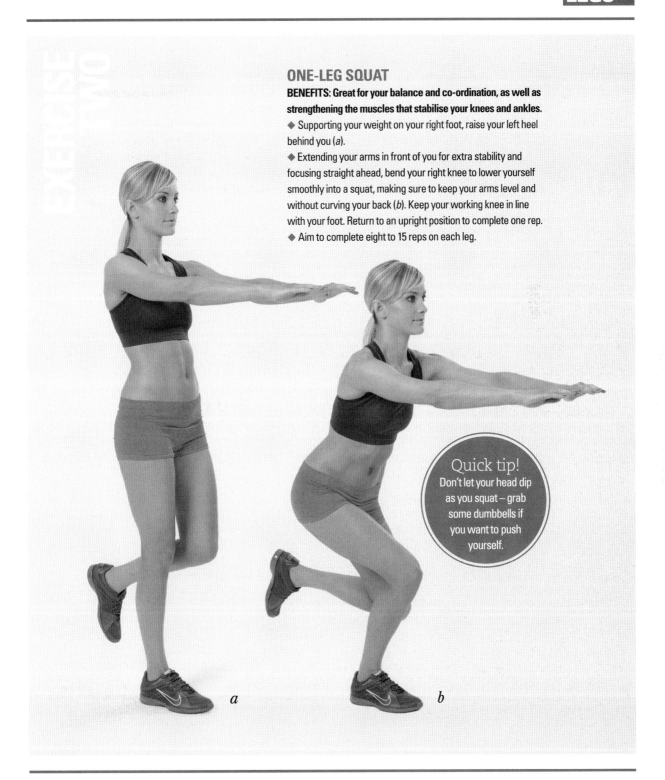

ONE-LEG SQUAT

BENEFITS: Great for your balance and co-ordination, as well as strengthening the muscles that stabilise your knees and ankles.

◆ Supporting your weight on your right foot, raise your left heel behind you (*a*).

◆ Extending your arms in front of you for extra stability and focusing straight ahead, bend your right knee to lower yourself smoothly into a squat, making sure to keep your arms level and without curving your back (*b*). Keep your working knee in line with your foot. Return to an upright position to complete one rep.

◆ Aim to complete eight to 15 reps on each leg.

Quick tip!
Don't let your head dip as you squat – grab some dumbbells if you want to push yourself.

a

b

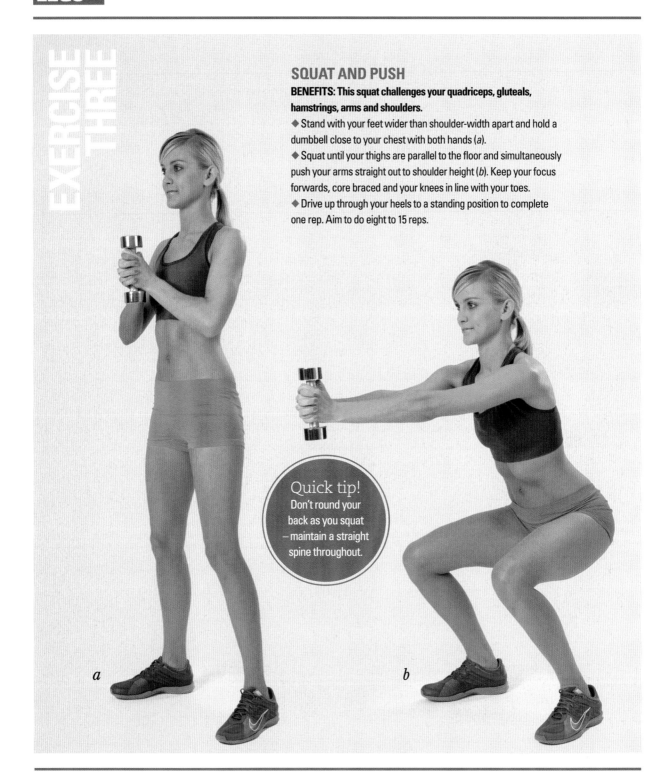

EXERCISE THREE

SQUAT AND PUSH

BENEFITS: This squat challenges your quadriceps, gluteals, hamstrings, arms and shoulders.

◆ Stand with your feet wider than shoulder-width apart and hold a dumbbell close to your chest with both hands (*a*).

◆ Squat until your thighs are parallel to the floor and simultaneously push your arms straight out to shoulder height (*b*). Keep your focus forwards, core braced and your knees in line with your toes.

◆ Drive up through your heels to a standing position to complete one rep. Aim to do eight to 15 reps.

Quick tip!
Don't round your back as you squat – maintain a straight spine throughout.

a

b

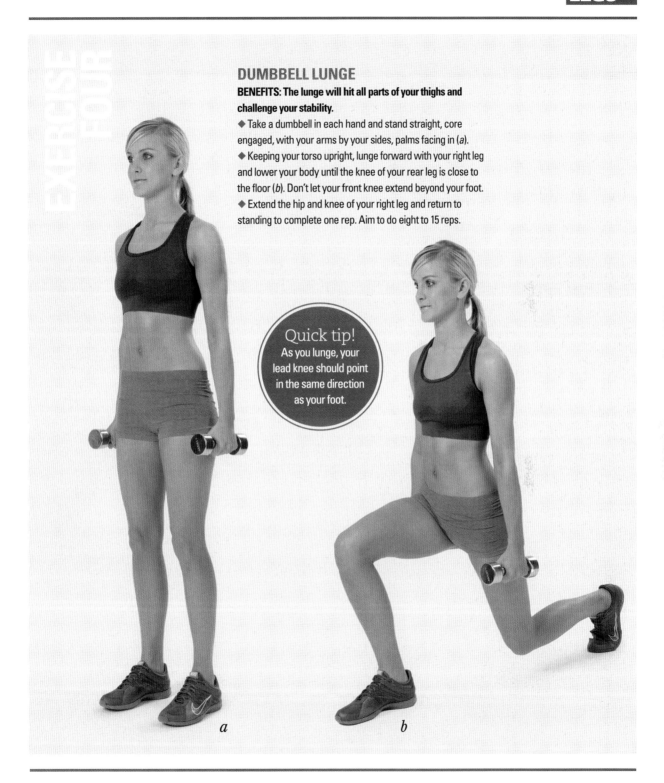

EXERCISE FOUR

DUMBBELL LUNGE

BENEFITS: The lunge will hit all parts of your thighs and challenge your stability.

◆ Take a dumbbell in each hand and stand straight, core engaged, with your arms by your sides, palms facing in (*a*).

◆ Keeping your torso upright, lunge forward with your right leg and lower your body until the knee of your rear leg is close to the floor (*b*). Don't let your front knee extend beyond your foot.

◆ Extend the hip and knee of your right leg and return to standing to complete one rep. Aim to do eight to 15 reps.

Quick tip!
As you lunge, your lead knee should point in the same direction as your foot.

a

b

EXERCISE FIVE

GYM BALL LEG CURL

BENEFITS: Uses your own body weight to challenge your hamstrings.

◆ Lie flat on your back with your lower legs on a gym ball, feet together. Your hands should be next to your hips.

◆ In a smooth movement, push your hips up so your body is in a straight line (*a*), then pull your heels towards you, rolling the ball towards your bum (*b*).

◆ Pause, then roll the ball back until your body is back in a straight line. Aim to do eight to 15 reps.

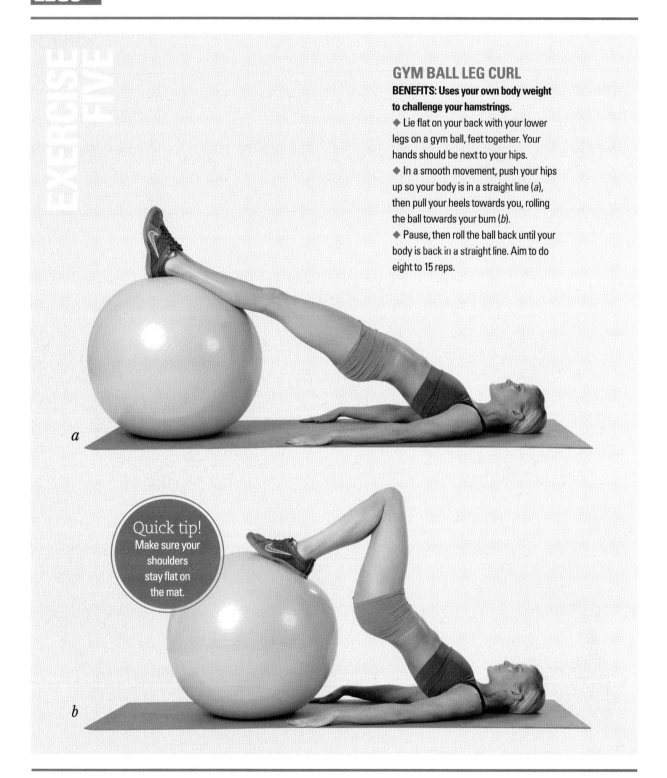

a

Quick tip!
Make sure your shoulders stay flat on the mat.

b

EXERCISE SIX

BOX JUMP

BENEFITS: A total body workout, great for your co-ordination and balance too.

◆ Stand just less than a foot away from your Step or box, feet shoulder-width apart and arms by your sides, knees slightly bent (*a*).

◆ Looking straight ahead, jump on to the Step, using your arms to power you (*b*). Hold for a count of one (*c*), then jump back down to complete one rep. Bend your knees slightly as you land. Aim to do eight to 15 reps.

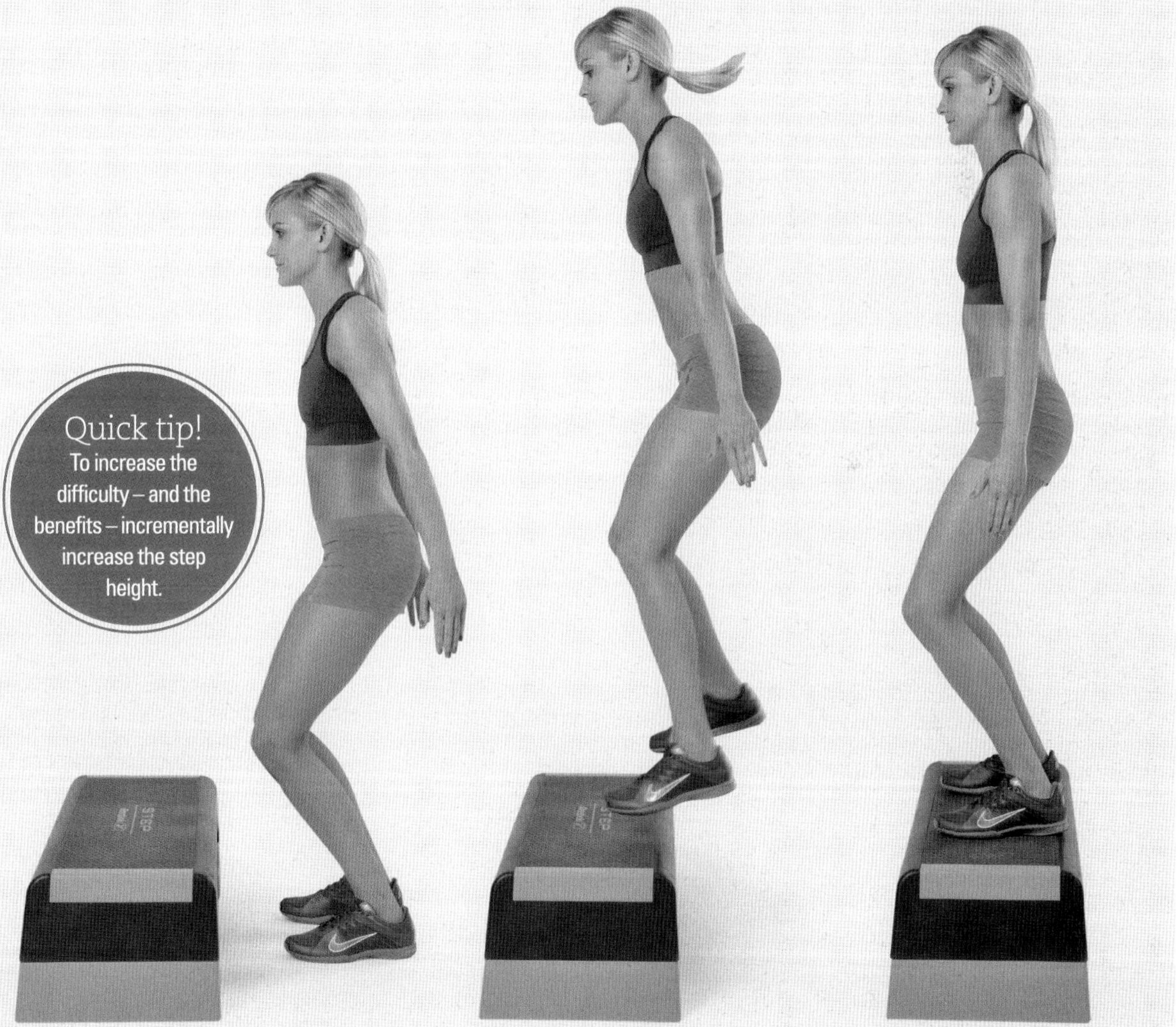

Quick tip!
To increase the difficulty – and the benefits – incrementally increase the step height.

a

b

c

EXERCISE SEVEN

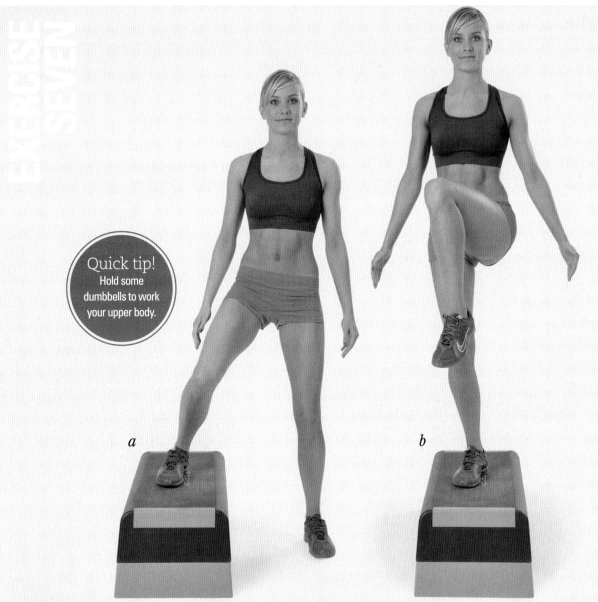

Quick tip!
Hold some dumbbells to work your upper body.

a

b

SIDE STEP-UP

BENEFITS: Challenge your gluteals from a new angle by introducing your inner-thigh muscles.

◆ Stand right side on to a Step, about a foot away from it.

◆ Dynamically step up (*a*), leading with your right leg, pushing up through your whole foot and keeping your body straight. As you do so, power your left knee up to waist height (*b*).

◆ Step down to the same side to complete one rep. Stand on the other side of the Step to repeat on the other side. Aim to do eight to 15 reps on each side.

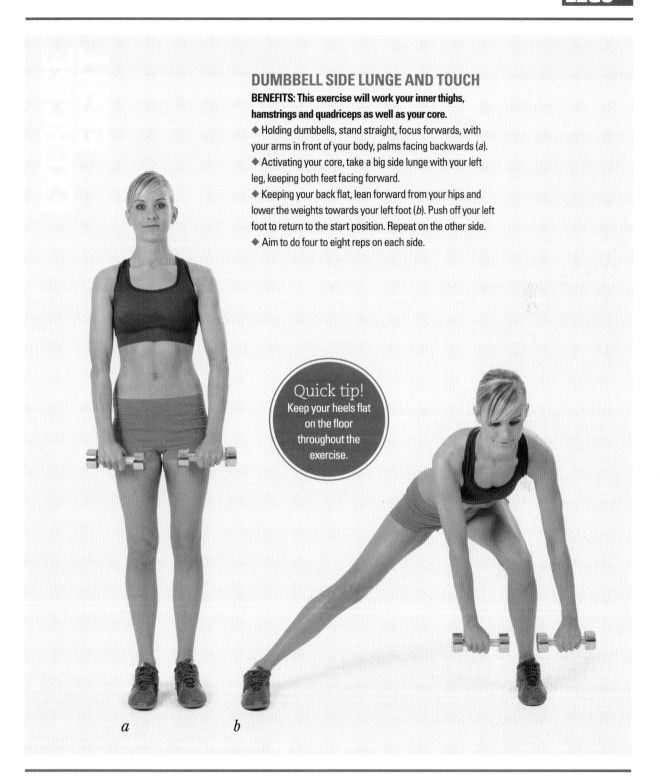

EXERCISE EIGHT

DUMBBELL SIDE LUNGE AND TOUCH

BENEFITS: This exercise will work your inner thighs, hamstrings and quadriceps as well as your core.

◆ Holding dumbbells, stand straight, focus forwards, with your arms in front of your body, palms facing backwards (*a*).

◆ Activating your core, take a big side lunge with your left leg, keeping both feet facing forward.

◆ Keeping your back flat, lean forward from your hips and lower the weights towards your left foot (*b*). Push off your left foot to return to the start position. Repeat on the other side.

◆ Aim to do four to eight reps on each side.

Quick tip!
Keep your heels flat on the floor throughout the exercise.

a   *b*

10-MINUTE LEGS WORKOUT
BEGINNER

An entry-level, no-kit circuit.

WHAT TO DO… Warm up properly, then try this dynamic circuit three times with 20 seconds' rest in between each exercise.

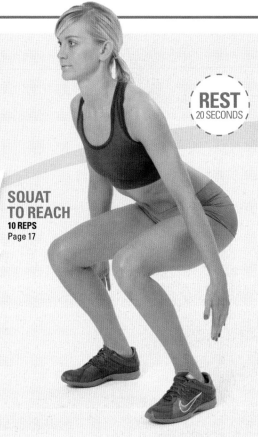

REST
20 SECONDS

1 **SQUAT TO REACH**
10 REPS
Page 17

EXERCISES	REPS/DURATION	PAGE
1. SQUAT TO REACH	10 REPS	17
REST	20 SECONDS	
2. ALTERNATING SPLIT DEADLIFT	10 REPS *(alternating sides)*	17
REST	20 SECONDS	
3. LUNGE TO FLYE	10 REPS *(alternating sides)*	17
REST	20 SECONDS	
4. LYING LATERAL LEG RAISE	8 REPS *(each side)*	64
REST	20 SECONDS	

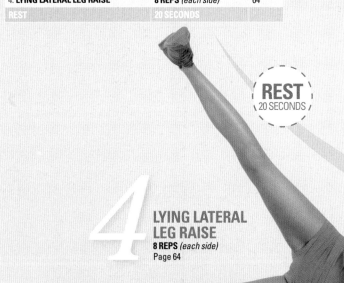

REST
20 SECONDS

4 **LYING LATERAL LEG RAISE**
8 REPS *(each side)*
Page 64

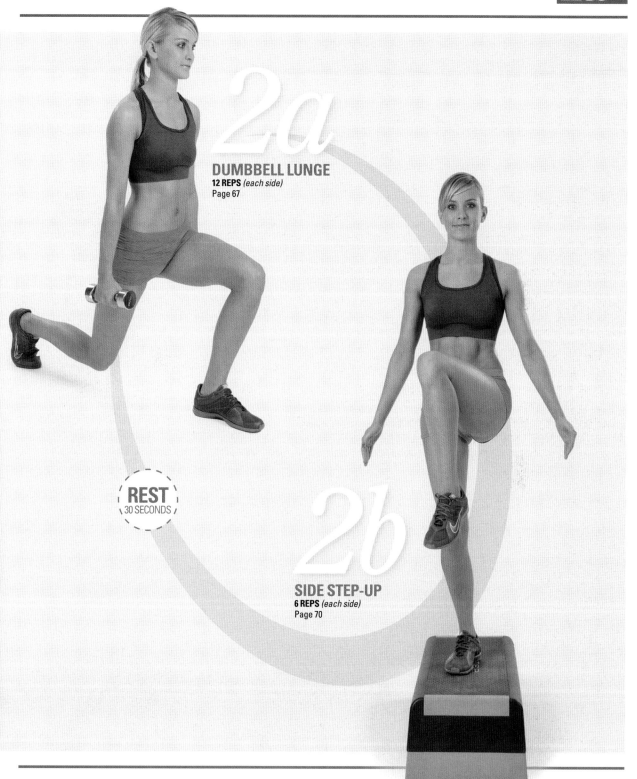

2a

DUMBBELL LUNGE
12 REPS *(each side)*
Page 67

REST
30 SECONDS

2b

SIDE STEP-UP
6 REPS *(each side)*
Page 70

10-MINUTE LEGS WORKOUT
INTERMEDIATE

A revved-up leg circuit for intermediates.

WHAT TO DO... Do exercise 1a immediately followed by 1b – that's one superset. Perform superset 1 three times, resting for 30 seconds between each set. Rest for one minute, then move on to do the same with superset 2. You'll need a Step or bench and dumbbells.

EXERCISES	REPS/DURATION	PAGE
1a. BOX JUMP	**12 REPS**	69
1b. ONE-LEG SQUAT	**6 REPS** *(each leg)*	65
REST	1 MINUTE	
2a. DUMBBELL LUNGE	**12 REPS** *(alternating sides)*	67
2b. SIDE STEP-UP	**6 REPS** *(each side)*	70

1a
BOX JUMP
12 REPS
Page 69

REST
30 SECONDS

1b
ONE-LEG SQUAT
6 REPS *(each side)*
Page 65

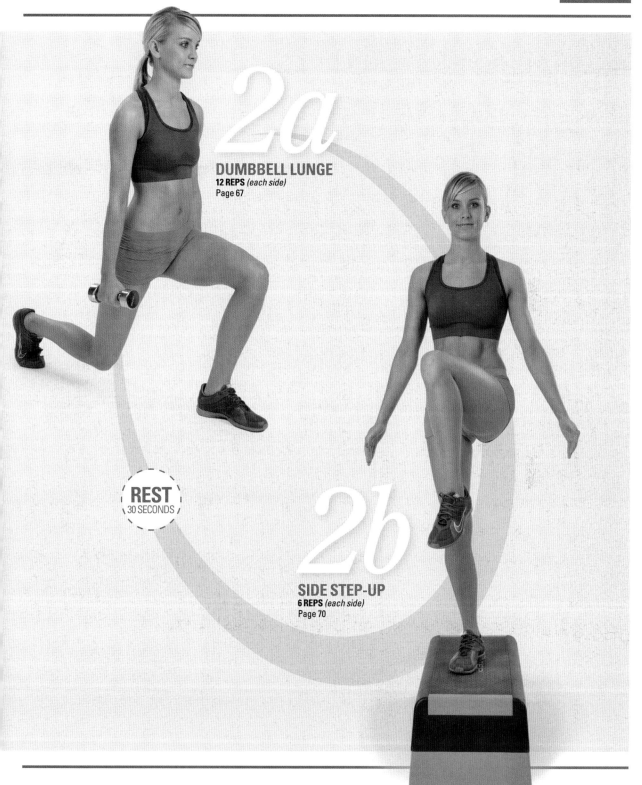

2a

DUMBBELL LUNGE
12 REPS *(each side)*
Page 67

REST
30 SECONDS

2b

SIDE STEP-UP
6 REPS *(each side)*
Page 70

10-MINUTE LEGS WORKOUT
ADVANCED

An intense circuit for exercise devotees.

WHAT TO DO… After a warm-up, do this circuit twice, resting for one minute in between. You'll need dumbbells and a gym ball.

EXERCISES	REPS/DURATION	PAGE
1. JUMPING JACKS	20 REPS	17
2. SQUAT AND PUSH	20 REPS	66
3. DUMBBELL SIDE LUNGE AND TOUCH	20 REPS *(alternating)*	71
4. DUMBBELL LUNGE	20 REPS *(alternating)*	67
5. GYM BALL LEG CURL	20 REPS	68
REST	1 MINUTE	

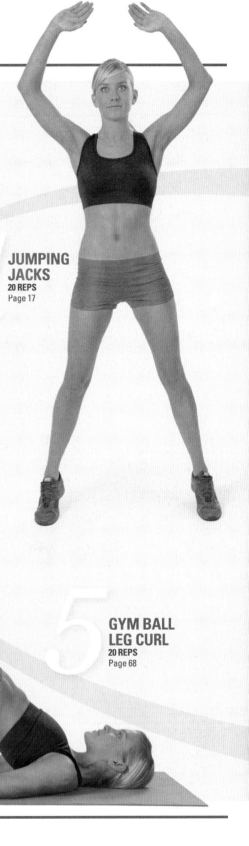

JUMPING JACKS
20 REPS
Page 17

REST
1 MINUTE

GYM BALL LEG CURL
20 REPS
Page 68

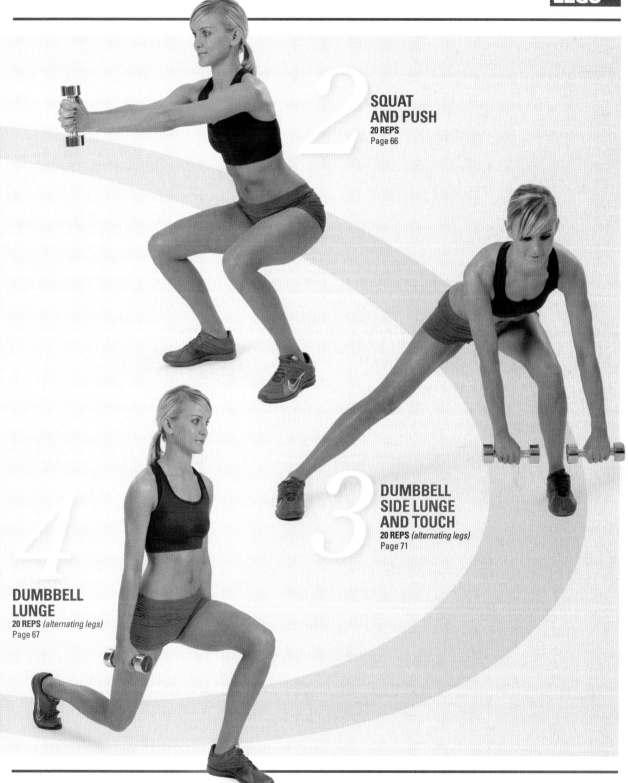

**SQUAT
AND PUSH**
20 REPS
Page 66

**DUMBBELL
SIDE LUNGE
AND TOUCH**
20 REPS *(alternating legs)*
Page 71

**DUMBBELL
LUNGE**
20 REPS *(alternating legs)*
Page 67

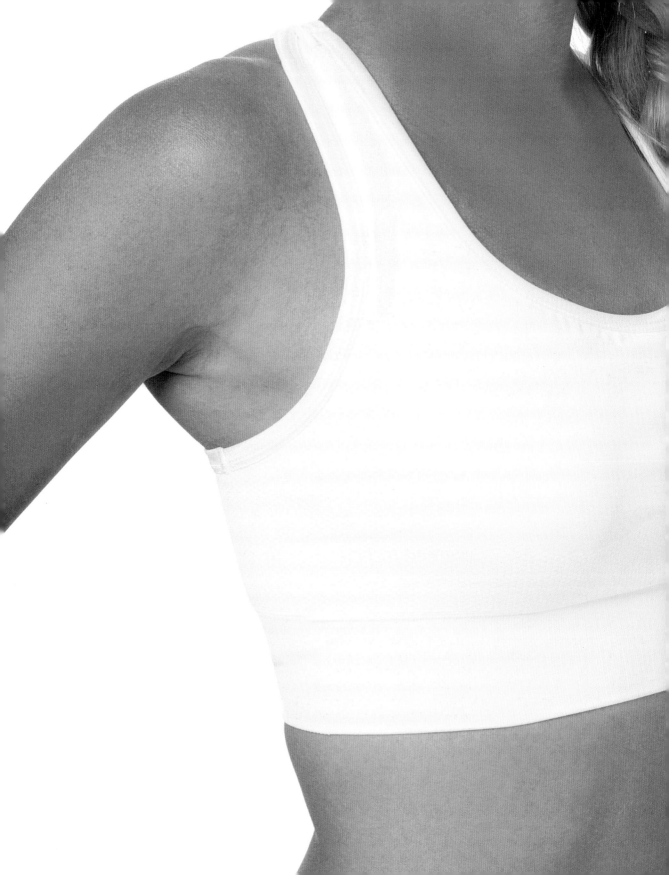

CHEST

The daily grind can really weaken your upper body. Driving a car and working at a computer constrict the chest muscles and lead to tension in the back. This set of exercises is designed to pep up your posture, open up your shoulders and tone up your pectorals and bust.

SIX WAYS TO A PERT BUST

1. You can't stop your boobs losing their pertness as you age, but you can minimise sagging by always wearing a sports bra when you exercise.

2. Work your chest and back in unison – strengthening your back and improving your posture will have untold benefits for the front of your body.

3. Slouching shortens your chest muscles. Whatever you're doing, wherever you are, regularly straighten your spine and check your shoulders are open.

4. The breaststroke is great for your pectorals (chest muscles). To boost the benefits, make sure you lift your upper body as your arms pull back.

5. Try some yoga chest openers – we recommend cobra, camel, fish and triangle poses.

6. Moisturise your neck and décolletage daily as you do your face.

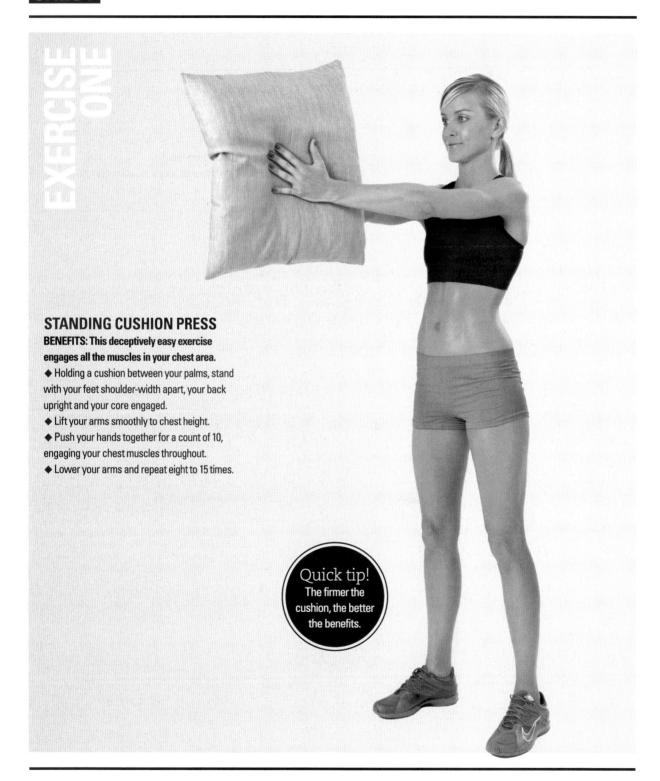

EXERCISE ONE

STANDING CUSHION PRESS

BENEFITS: This deceptively easy exercise engages all the muscles in your chest area.

◆ Holding a cushion between your palms, stand with your feet shoulder-width apart, your back upright and your core engaged.

◆ Lift your arms smoothly to chest height.

◆ Push your hands together for a count of 10, engaging your chest muscles throughout.

◆ Lower your arms and repeat eight to 15 times.

Quick tip!
The firmer the cushion, the better the benefits.

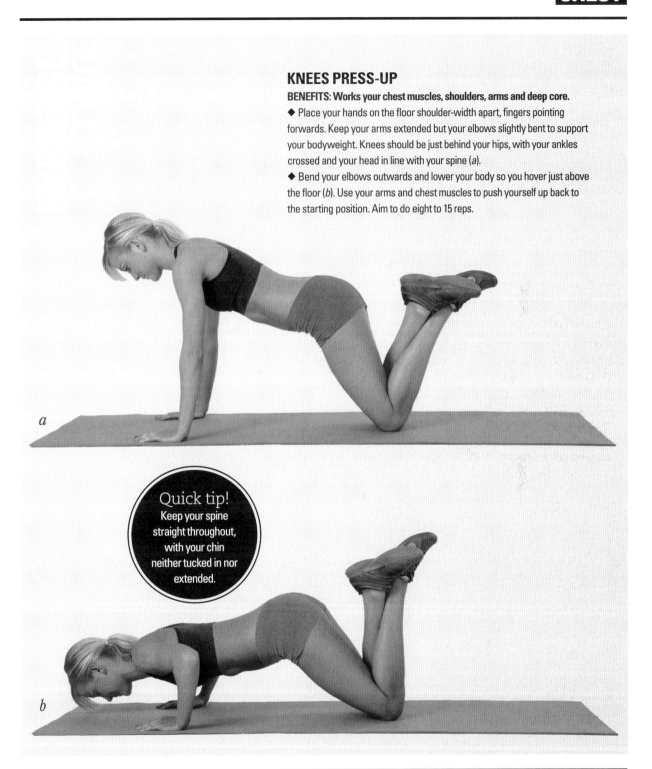

KNEES PRESS-UP

BENEFITS: Works your chest muscles, shoulders, arms and deep core.

◆ Place your hands on the floor shoulder-width apart, fingers pointing forwards. Keep your arms extended but your elbows slightly bent to support your bodyweight. Knees should be just behind your hips, with your ankles crossed and your head in line with your spine (*a*).

◆ Bend your elbows outwards and lower your body so you hover just above the floor (*b*). Use your arms and chest muscles to push yourself up back to the starting position. Aim to do eight to 15 reps.

a

Quick tip!
Keep your spine straight throughout, with your chin neither tucked in nor extended.

b

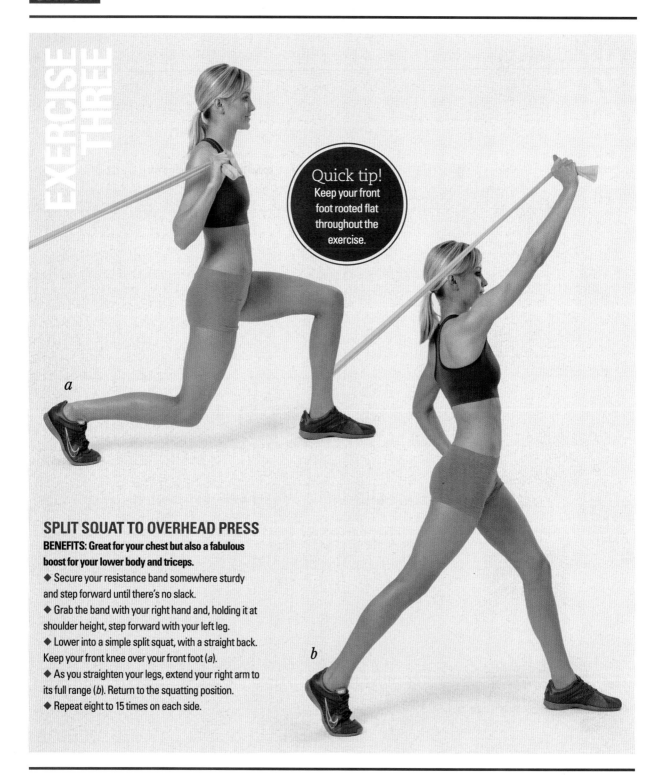

EXERCISE THREE

a

b

Quick tip!
Keep your front foot rooted flat throughout the exercise.

SPLIT SQUAT TO OVERHEAD PRESS

BENEFITS: Great for your chest but also a fabulous boost for your lower body and triceps.

◆ Secure your resistance band somewhere sturdy and step forward until there's no slack.

◆ Grab the band with your right hand and, holding it at shoulder height, step forward with your left leg.

◆ Lower into a simple split squat, with a straight back. Keep your front knee over your front foot (*a*).

◆ As you straighten your legs, extend your right arm to its full range (*b*). Return to the squatting position.

◆ Repeat eight to 15 times on each side.

EXERCISE FOUR

SHADOW BOXING

BENEFITS: Primes your cardiovascular system, tests your agility and opens up your chest.

◆ With your left foot placed about a metre in front of your right, bring your hands up to the guard position, elbows close to the body. Flex your right heel from the floor (*a*).

◆ Throw out a range of punches such as jabs (straight out) (*b*), hooks (from the side) and uppercuts (up) (*c*).

◆ Use your whole body in each punch, pushing off your legs and twisting your shoulders and torso as you punch.

◆ Keep it fast and fluid to get your heart pumping. Aim to keep boxing for one to two minutes.

Quick tip!
Move around quickly to raise your heart rate.

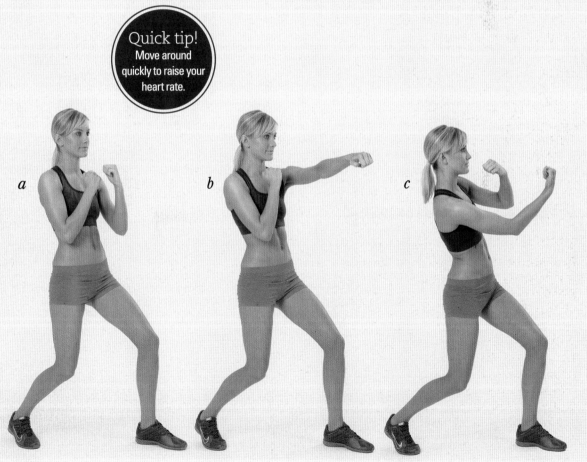

a

b

c

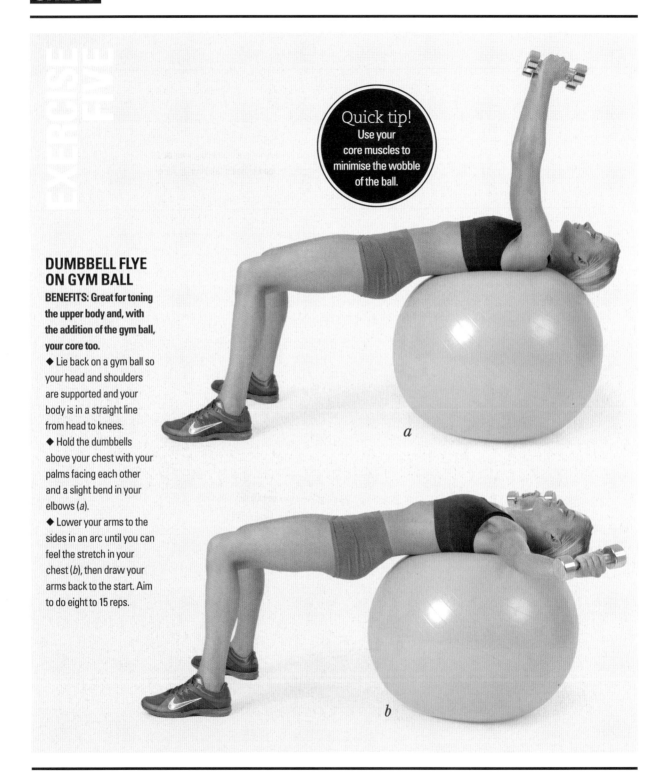

EXERCISE FIVE

Quick tip!
Use your core muscles to minimise the wobble of the ball.

DUMBBELL FLYE ON GYM BALL

BENEFITS: Great for toning the upper body and, with the addition of the gym ball, your core too.

◆ Lie back on a gym ball so your head and shoulders are supported and your body is in a straight line from head to knees.

◆ Hold the dumbbells above your chest with your palms facing each other and a slight bend in your elbows (*a*).

◆ Lower your arms to the sides in an arc until you can feel the stretch in your chest (*b*), then draw your arms back to the start. Aim to do eight to 15 reps.

a

b

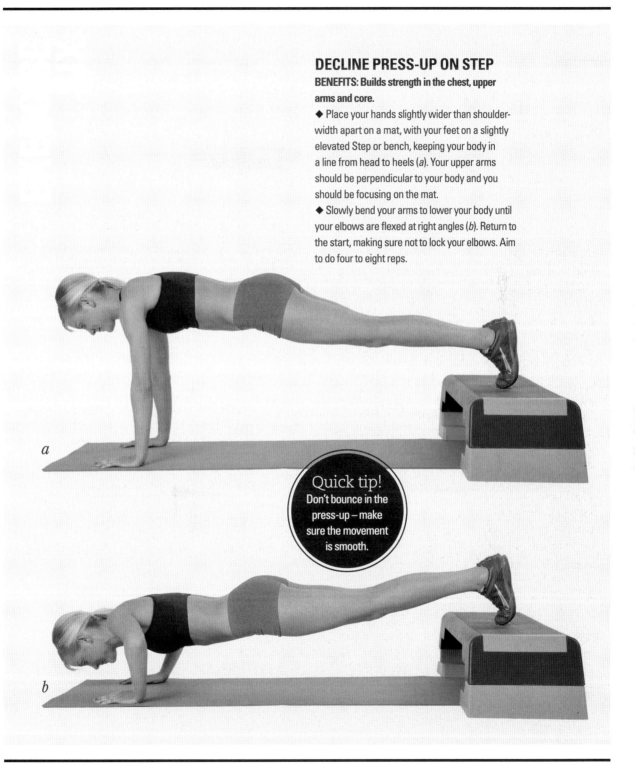

DECLINE PRESS-UP ON STEP

BENEFITS: Builds strength in the chest, upper arms and core.

◆ Place your hands slightly wider than shoulder-width apart on a mat, with your feet on a slightly elevated Step or bench, keeping your body in a line from head to heels (*a*). Your upper arms should be perpendicular to your body and you should be focusing on the mat.

◆ Slowly bend your arms to lower your body until your elbows are flexed at right angles (*b*). Return to the start, making sure not to lock your elbows. Aim to do four to eight reps.

a

Quick tip!
Don't bounce in the press-up – make sure the movement is smooth.

b

EXERCISE SEVEN

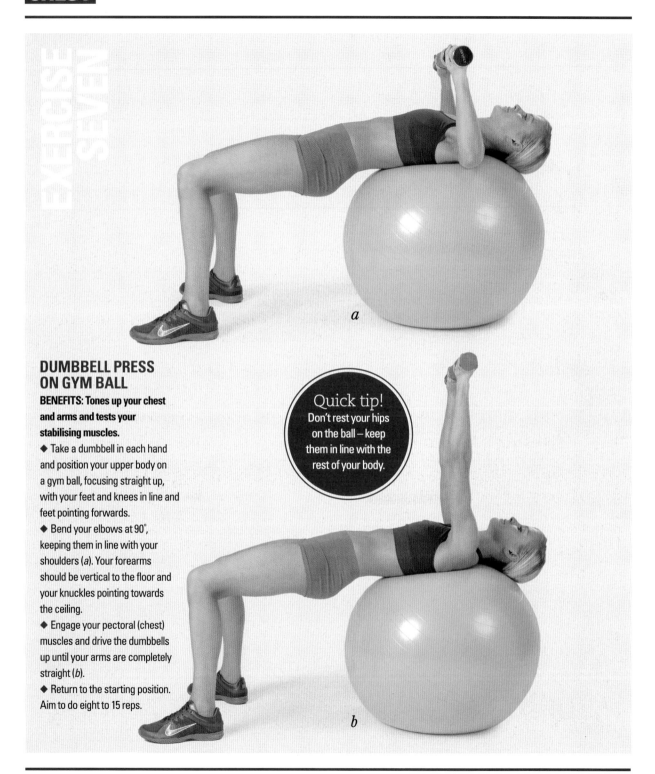

a

DUMBBELL PRESS ON GYM BALL

BENEFITS: Tones up your chest and arms and tests your stabilising muscles.

◆ Take a dumbbell in each hand and position your upper body on a gym ball, focusing straight up, with your feet and knees in line and feet pointing forwards.

◆ Bend your elbows at 90°, keeping them in line with your shoulders (*a*). Your forearms should be vertical to the floor and your knuckles pointing towards the ceiling.

◆ Engage your pectoral (chest) muscles and drive the dumbbells up until your arms are completely straight (*b*).

◆ Return to the starting position. Aim to do eight to 15 reps.

Quick tip!
Don't rest your hips on the ball – keep them in line with the rest of your body.

b

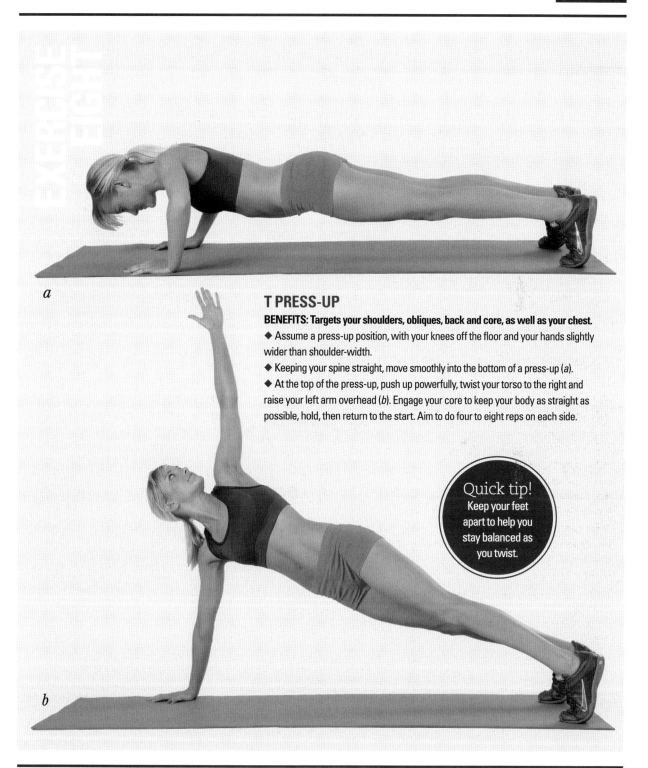

EXERCISE EIGHT

a

T PRESS-UP

BENEFITS: Targets your shoulders, obliques, back and core, as well as your chest.

◆ Assume a press-up position, with your knees off the floor and your hands slightly wider than shoulder-width.

◆ Keeping your spine straight, move smoothly into the bottom of a press-up (*a*).

◆ At the top of the press-up, push up powerfully, twist your torso to the right and raise your left arm overhead (*b*). Engage your core to keep your body as straight as possible, hold, then return to the start. Aim to do four to eight reps on each side.

Quick tip!
Keep your feet apart to help you stay balanced as you twist.

b

10-MINUTE CHEST WORKOUT
BEGINNER

An entry-level chest circuit.

WHAT TO DO… You don't need any equipment for this one. After your warm-up, simply perform the circuit three times, resting for one minute after each circuit. Do as many reps as you can in the time stated, keeping the pace high but controlled.

EXERCISES	DURATION	PAGE
1. SIDE LUNGE WITH TWIST	30 SECONDS *(alternating)*	17
2. KNEES PRESS-UP	30 SECONDS	81
REST	30 SECONDS	
3. SQUAT TO REACH	30 SECONDS	17
4. STANDING CUSHION PRESS	30 SECONDS	80
REST	1 MINUTE	

REST
1 MINUTE

STANDING CUSHION PRESS
30 SECONDS
Page 80

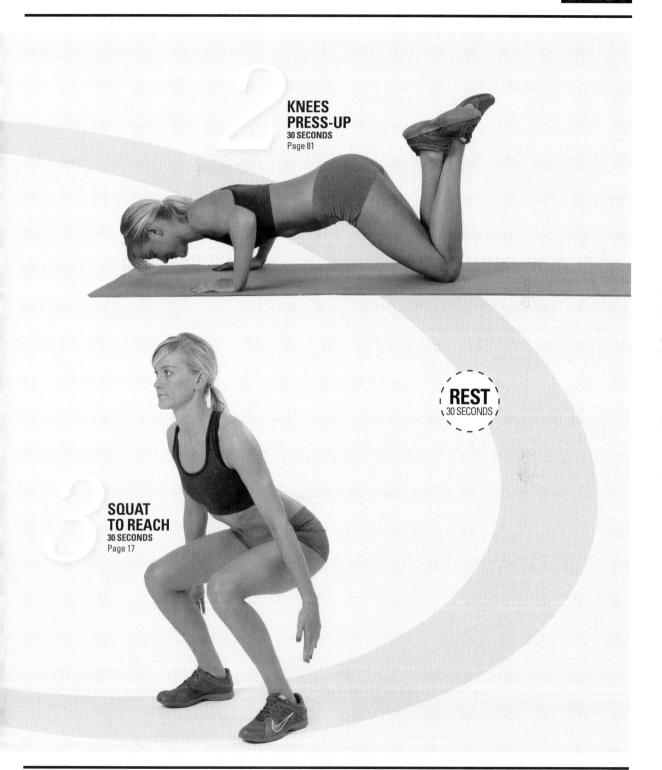

2

**KNEES
PRESS-UP**
30 SECONDS
Page 81

REST
30 SECONDS

3

**SQUAT
TO REACH**
30 SECONDS
Page 17

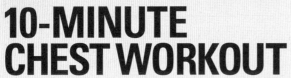

10-MINUTE CHEST WORKOUT
INTERMEDIATE

A duo of supersets for intermediates.

WHAT TO DO… Grab your dumbbells and a gym ball for this powerful circuit. Perform exercise 1a followed immediately by 1b — that's one superset. Do superset 1 three times, resting for 30 seconds between each set. Rest for one minute before doing the same with superset 2.

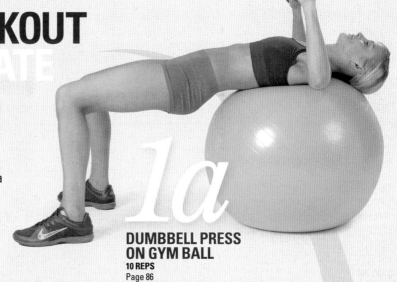

1a

DUMBBELL PRESS ON GYM BALL
10 REPS
Page 86

EXERCISES	REPS/DURATION	PAGE
1a. DUMBBELL PRESS ON GYM BALL	10 REPS	86
1b. DUMBBELL FLYE ON GYM BALL	10 REPS	84
REST	1 MINUTE	
2a. DECLINE PRESS-UP ON STEP	TO FAILURE	85
2b. STANDING CUSHION PRESS	30 SECONDS	80

REST
30 SECONDS

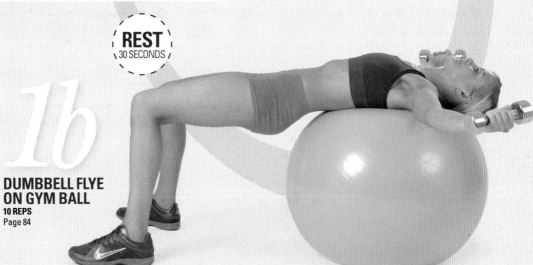

1b

DUMBBELL FLYE ON GYM BALL
10 REPS
Page 84

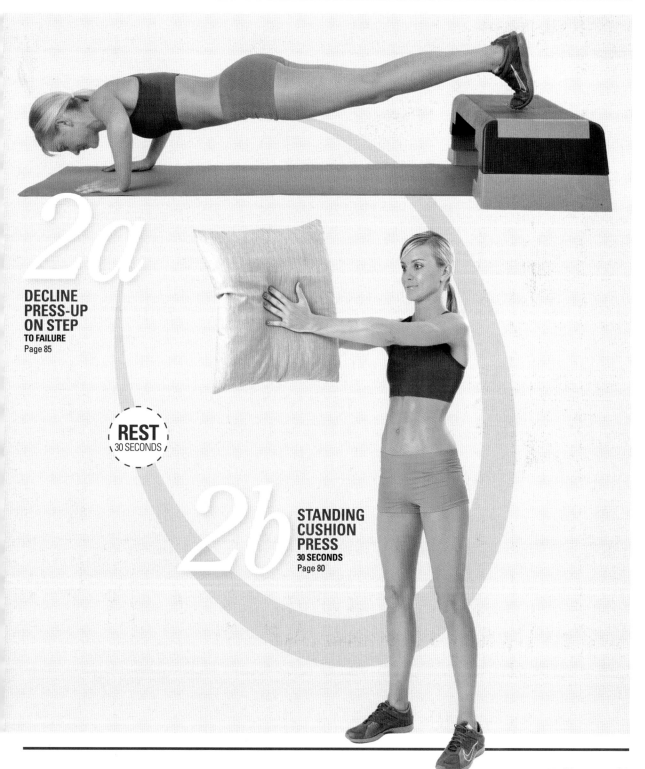

2a

**DECLINE
PRESS-UP
ON STEP**
TO FAILURE
Page 85

REST
30 SECONDS

2b

**STANDING
CUSHION
PRESS**
30 SECONDS
Page 80

10-MINUTE CHEST WORKOUT

An advanced challenge for your chest.

WHAT TO DO… Perform this circuit three times over. Don't rest between exercises, but do allow yourself one minute's respite between circuits. Keep the pace as high as you can manage without compromising good form on any of the exercises.

SQUAT TO REACH
30 SECONDS
Page 17

EXERCISES	DURATION	PAGE
1. SQUAT TO REACH	30 SECONDS	17
2. T PRESS-UP	30 SECONDS *(alternating)*	87
3. SPLIT SQUAT TO OVERHEAD PRESS (RIGHT)	30 SECONDS	82
4. SPLIT SQUAT TO OVERHEAD PRESS (LEFT)	30 SECONDS	82
5. SHADOW BOXING	30 SECONDS	83
REST	1 MINUTE	

REST
1 MINUTE

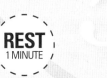
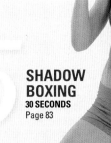

SHADOW BOXING
30 SECONDS
Page 83

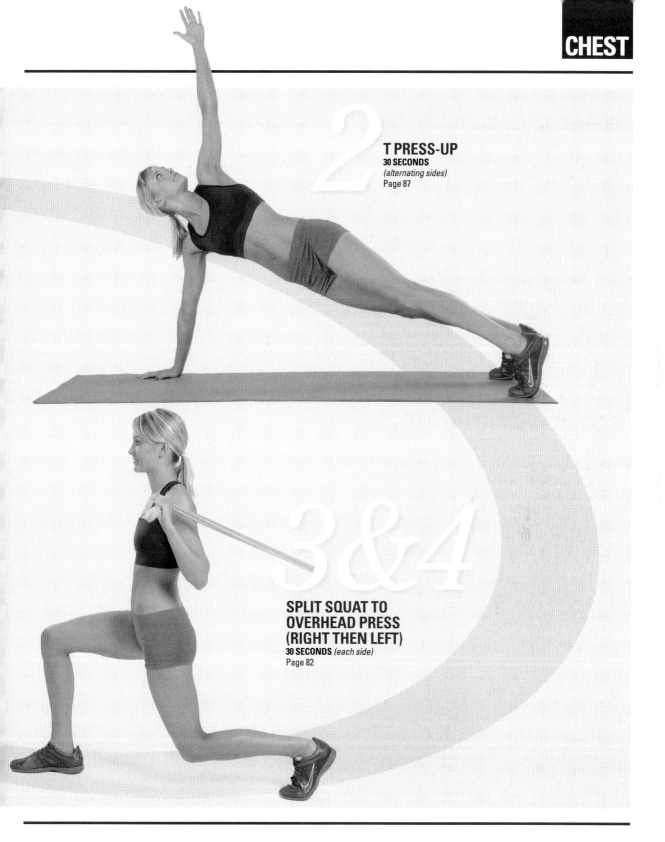

2
T PRESS-UP
30 SECONDS
(alternating sides)
Page 87

3 & 4
**SPLIT SQUAT TO
OVERHEAD PRESS
(RIGHT THEN LEFT)**
30 SECONDS *(each side)*
Page 82

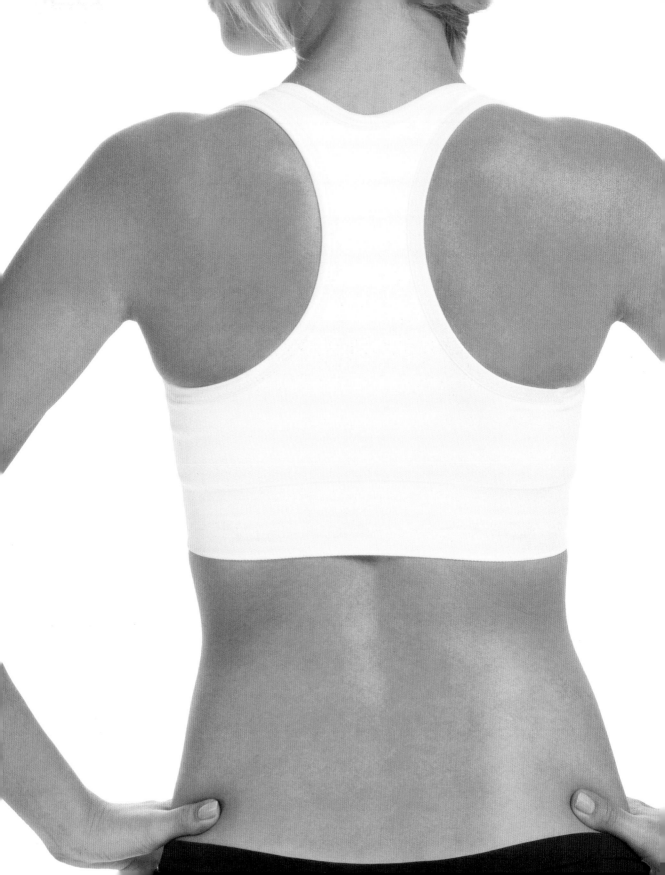

BACK

You can't see it without contortions in a mirror. But devote time to your back and you'll not only gain backless-dress confidence, you'll improve posture and prevent injury.

SIX WAYS TO A SEXY BACK

1. Pilates is the ultimate posture exercise and fab for toning your back muscles.

2. During the day, realign your upper body to engage your back muscles – rotate your shoulders up and around until you bring the blades together.

3. Book a regular deep-tissue massage to target tension in your back and improve your flexibility during exercise.

4. Include the rowing machine in your gym cardio regime. To boost your back, bend forwards from the hips rather than curving your spine as you row.

5. If you spend time hunched over a computer or steering wheel, take regular breaks to open up the front of your body. Do some roll-downs and roll-ups to activate your spine.

6. Don't neglect your back in your beauty regime – ask your partner to exfoliate and moisturise the bits you can't reach.

EXERCISE ONE

DUMBBELL BENT-OVER ROW

BENEFITS: Great for the sets of muscles that criss-cross your upper back.

◆ Dumbbells in hands, stand with your feet shoulder-width apart, keeping a bend in your knees. Bend forwards from the hips, letting your arms hang down beneath your shoulders, palms facing in (*a*).

◆ Holding your torso still, take a deep breath in and pull the dumbbells up to chest height, keeping your elbows close to your body and making sure they don't flail outwards (*b*). Pause briefly before returning to the start. Try to do eight to 15 reps.

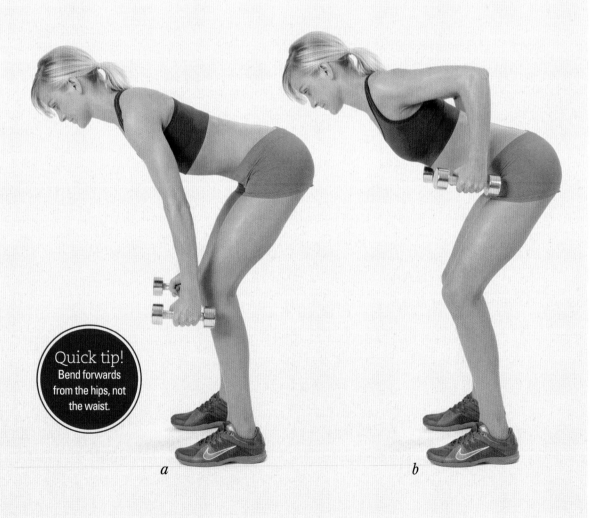

Quick tip!
Bend forwards from the hips, not the waist.

a　　　　　*b*

DUMBBELL BENT-OVER FLYE

BENEFITS: Target your back by taking arm strength out of the equation.

◆ Dumbbells in hands, stand with your feet shoulder-width apart, keeping a slight bend in your elbows. Bend forwards at the hips, focusing on the floor, and bring the weights together, palms facing in (*a*).

◆ Smoothly raise your arms out to the sides until they're level with your shoulders, keeping the slight bend in your elbows. Squeeze your shoulderblades slowly together (*b*), then lower your arms. Try to do eight to 15 reps.

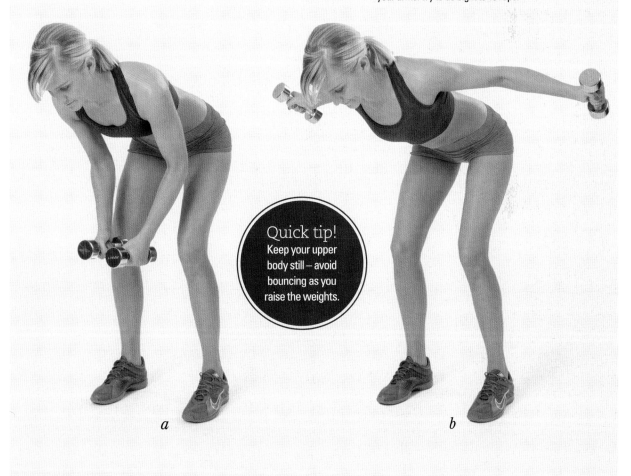

Quick tip!
Keep your upper body still – avoid bouncing as you raise the weights.

a

b

EXERCISE THREE

FOUR-POINT BOX

BENEFITS: Fabulous for your deep core and the stabilising muscles around your spine.

◆ Kneel on all fours, looking at the floor. Your hands should be positioned under your shoulders, knees under your hips and your spine straight (*a*).

◆ Switching on your core muscles, extend your right arm and left leg out to same height. Avoid shifting to one side or raising your head as you move (*b*). Hold and return to the start position, then swap sides and repeat. Aim to do four to six reps on each side.

Quick tip!
During the extension, keep your body in a straight line from foot to fingertips.

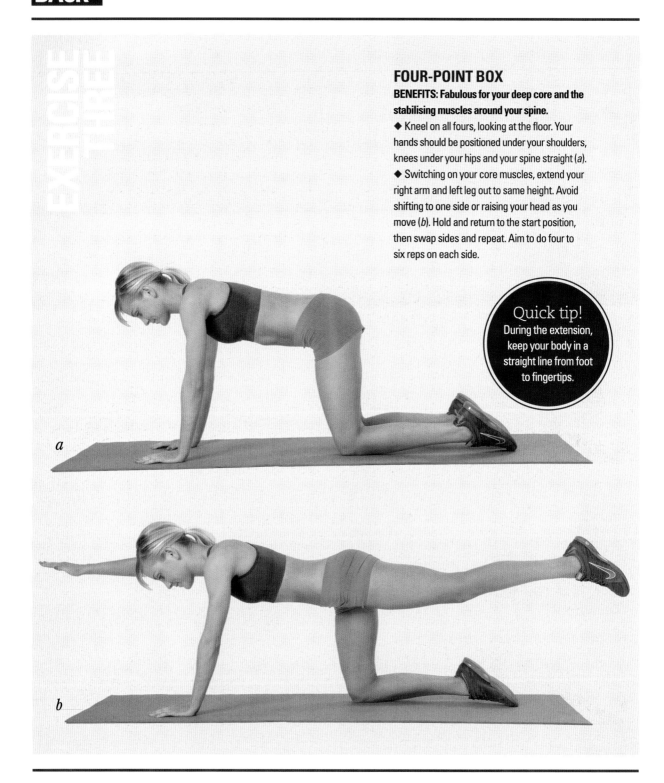

a

b

EXERCISE FOUR

DORSAL RAISE WITH SHOULDER ROTATION

BENEFITS: This move will strengthen your lower back and increase flexibility in your shoulders, back and chest.

◆ Lie face-down on a mat, looking down but with your chin in line with your spine, rather than tucked in. Extend your arms to the sides so they're in line with your shoulders, palms facing down, hovering just above the floor (*a*).

◆ Engage your abdominals and lift your upper body gently from the mat, turning your palms out.

◆ When you've reached your full range, twist your hands back so your thumbs point towards the ceiling and squeeze your shoulderblades together (*b*). Hold and return to start. Aim to do eight to 15 reps.

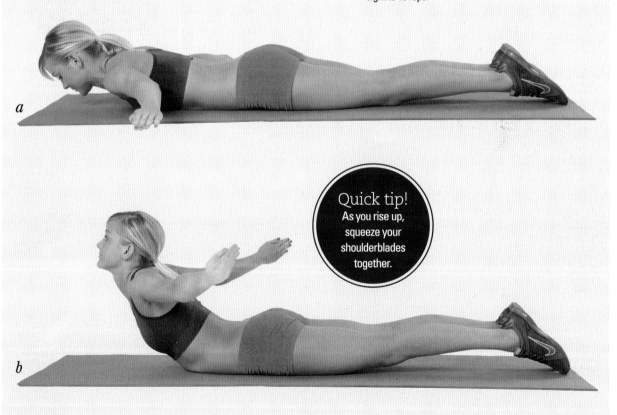

a

b

Quick tip!
As you rise up, squeeze your shoulderblades together.

EXERCISE FIVE

AQUAMAN

BENEFITS: This Pilates-style exercise works all your posterior muscles from your shoulders to your hamstrings.

◆ Lie face-down on a mat with your arms stretched out in front of you, hands in line with your shoulders, and your toes pointed.

◆ Keeping your pubic bone pressed down and your bum squeezed, gently lift your upper back, head and legs slightly off the mat.

◆ Keeping your focus forwards, simultaneously extend your right arm and left leg a little higher (*a*).

◆ Alternate arms and legs slowly in a swimming motion (*b*). Aim to do six to 10 reps on each side.

Quick tip!
To prevent compression in your spine, avoid lifting yourself too high off the mat.

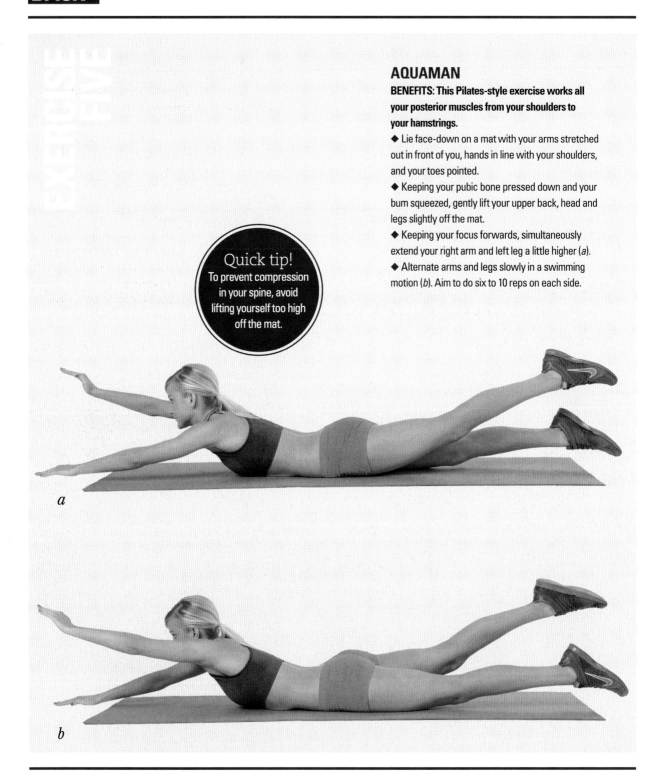

a

b

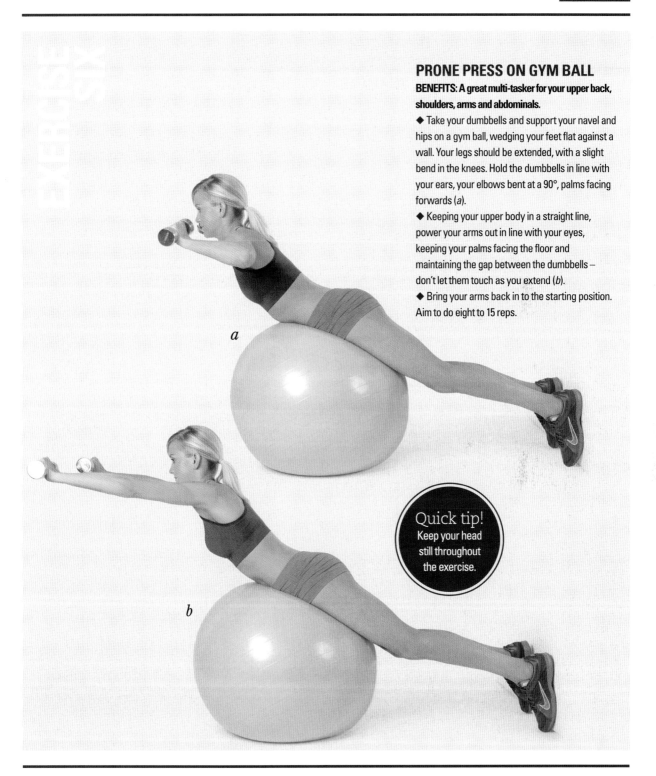

PRONE PRESS ON GYM BALL

BENEFITS: A great multi-tasker for your upper back, shoulders, arms and abdominals.

◆ Take your dumbbells and support your navel and hips on a gym ball, wedging your feet flat against a wall. Your legs should be extended, with a slight bend in the knees. Hold the dumbbells in line with your ears, your elbows bent at a 90°, palms facing forwards (*a*).

◆ Keeping your upper body in a straight line, power your arms out in line with your eyes, keeping your palms facing the floor and maintaining the gap between the dumbbells – don't let them touch as you extend (*b*).

◆ Bring your arms back in to the starting position. Aim to do eight to 15 reps.

a

b

Quick tip!
Keep your head still throughout the exercise.

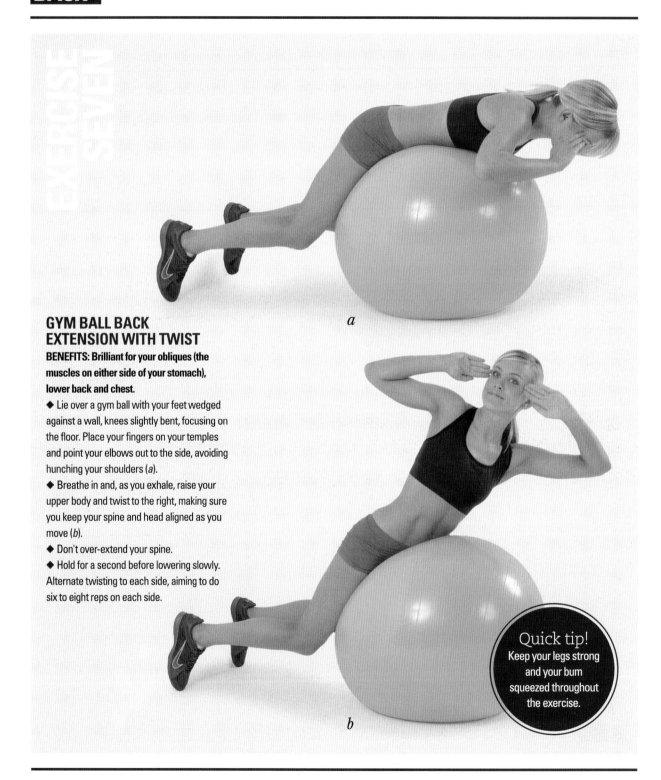

EXERCISE SEVEN

a

GYM BALL BACK EXTENSION WITH TWIST

BENEFITS: Brilliant for your obliques (the muscles on either side of your stomach), lower back and chest.

◆ Lie over a gym ball with your feet wedged against a wall, knees slightly bent, focusing on the floor. Place your fingers on your temples and point your elbows out to the side, avoiding hunching your shoulders (*a*).

◆ Breathe in and, as you exhale, raise your upper body and twist to the right, making sure you keep your spine and head aligned as you move (*b*).

◆ Don't over-extend your spine.

◆ Hold for a second before lowering slowly. Alternate twisting to each side, aiming to do six to eight reps on each side.

Quick tip!
Keep your legs strong and your bum squeezed throughout the exercise.

b

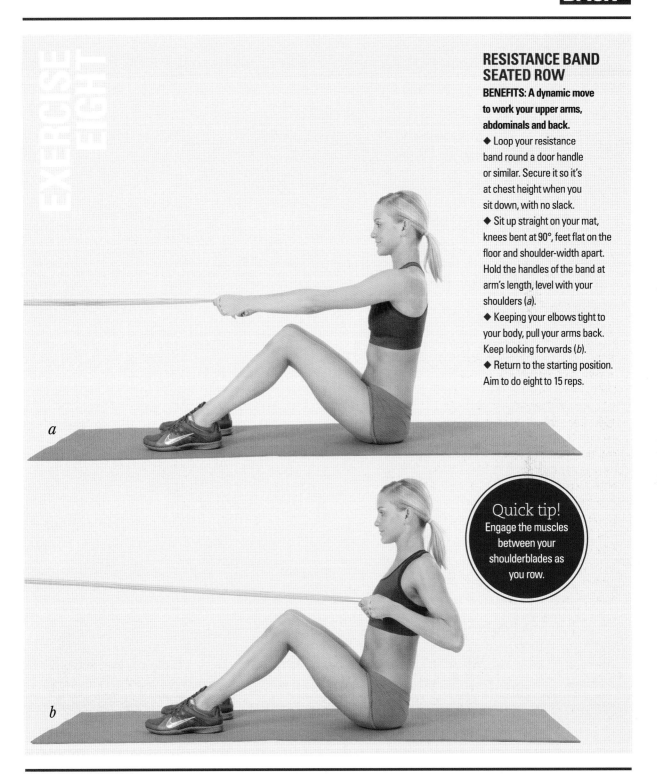

EXERCISE EIGHT

a

b

RESISTANCE BAND SEATED ROW

BENEFITS: A dynamic move to work your upper arms, abdominals and back.

◆ Loop your resistance band round a door handle or similar. Secure it so it's at chest height when you sit down, with no slack.

◆ Sit up straight on your mat, knees bent at 90°, feet flat on the floor and shoulder-width apart. Hold the handles of the band at arm's length, level with your shoulders (*a*).

◆ Keeping your elbows tight to your body, pull your arms back. Keep looking forwards (*b*).

◆ Return to the starting position. Aim to do eight to 15 reps.

Quick tip!
Engage the muscles between your shoulderblades as you row.

10-MINUTE BACK WORKOUT
BEGINNER

A simple back circuit for beginners.

WHAT TO DO... Once you've warmed up, perform this circuit twice. You'll need your resistance band so prepare it beforehand.

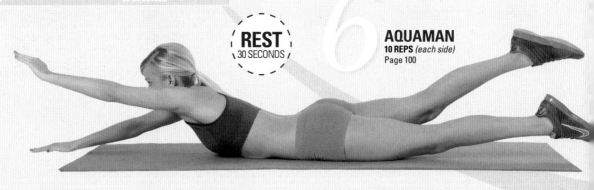

1 RESISTANCE BAND SEATED ROW
15 REPS
Page 103

EXERCISES	REPS	PAGE
1. RESISTANCE BAND SEATED ROW	15 REPS	103
2. FOUR-POINT BOX	10 REPS *(alternating)*	98
REST	30 SECONDS	
3. RESISTANCE BAND SEATED ROW	10 REPS	103
4. DORSAL RAISE WITH SHOULDER ROTATION	5 REPS *(hold each for a count of four)*	99
REST	30 SECONDS	
5. RESISTANCE BAND SEATED ROW	8 REPS	103
6. AQUAMAN	10 REPS *(each side)*	100
REST	30 SECONDS	

REST 30 SECONDS

6 AQUAMAN
10 REPS *(each side)*
Page 100

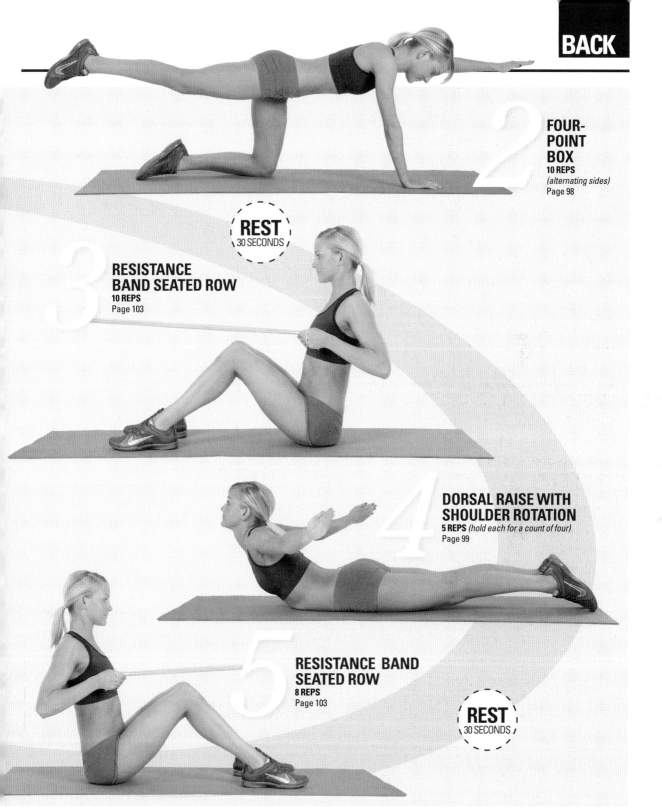

FOUR-POINT BOX
10 REPS
(alternating sides)
Page 98

REST
30 SECONDS

RESISTANCE BAND SEATED ROW
10 REPS
Page 103

DORSAL RAISE WITH SHOULDER ROTATION
5 REPS *(hold each for a count of four)*
Page 99

RESISTANCE BAND SEATED ROW
8 REPS
Page 103

REST
30 SECONDS

10-MINUTE BACK WORKOUT
INTERMEDIATE

Push yourself a little further with this intermediate challenge.

WHAT TO DO… Do this circuit twice. Make sure your dumbbells and gym ball are ready, and don't forget to stretch out afterwards.

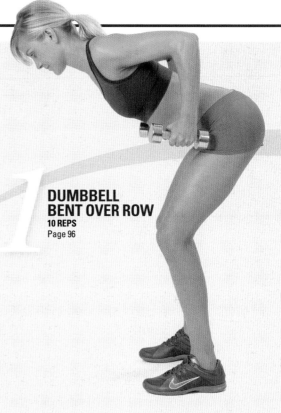

1

DUMBBELL BENT OVER ROW
10 REPS
Page 96

EXERCISES	REPS/DURATION	PAGE
1. DUMBBELL BENT OVER ROW	10 REPS	96
2. PRONE PRESS ON GYM BALL	10 REPS	101
3. DORSAL RAISE WITH SHOULDER ROTATION	10 REPS	99
REST	1 MINUTE	
4. DUMBBELL BENT OVER FLYE	10 REPS	97
5. GYM BALL BACK EXTENSION WITH TWIST	10 REPS *(alternating)*	102
6. FOUR-POINT BOX	6 REPS *(alternating – hold each for a count of four)*	98
REST	1 MINUTE	

REST
1 MINUTE

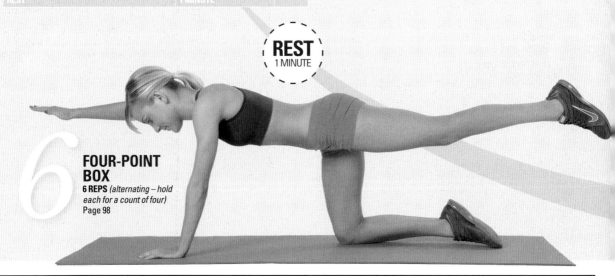

6

FOUR-POINT BOX
6 REPS *(alternating – hold each for a count of four)*
Page 98

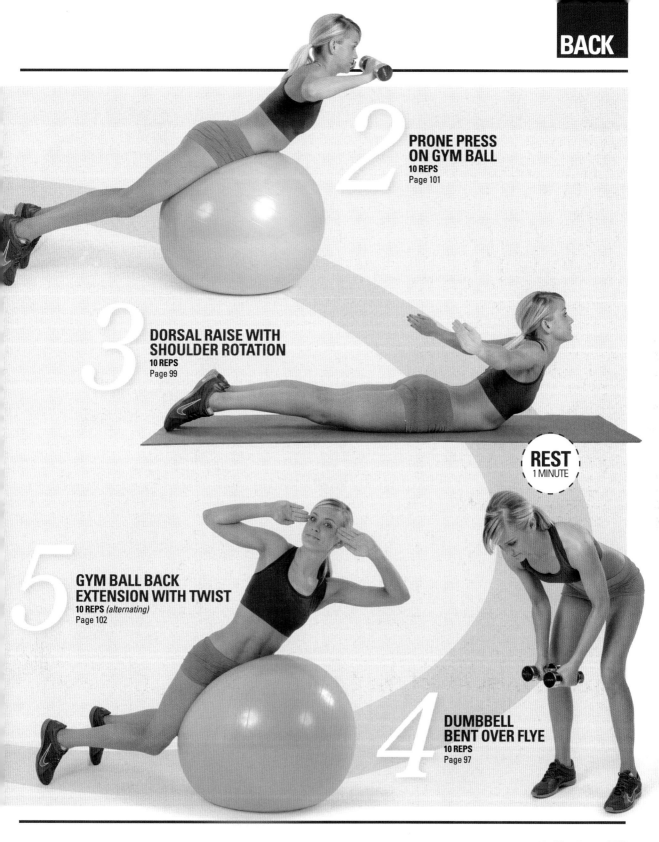

2

**PRONE PRESS
ON GYM BALL**
10 REPS
Page 101

3

**DORSAL RAISE WITH
SHOULDER ROTATION**
10 REPS
Page 99

REST
1 MINUTE

5

**GYM BALL BACK
EXTENSION WITH TWIST**
10 REPS (alternating)
Page 102

4

**DUMBBELL
BENT OVER FLYE**
10 REPS
Page 97

10-MINUTE BACK WORKOUT
ADVANCED

An advanced circuit for regular gym-goers.

WHAT TO DO... Perform exercise 1a followed immediately by exercise 1b – that's one superset. Do superset 1 three times, resting for 40 seconds between each. Then rest for one minute and do the same with superset 2.

EXERCISES	REPS/DURATION	PAGE
1a. DUMBBELL BENT-OVER ROW	**12 REPS**	96
1b. DUMBBELL BENT-OVER FLYE	**12 REPS**	97
REST	**1 MINUTE**	
2a. PRONE PRESS ON GYM BALL	**12 REPS**	101
2b. GYM BALL BACK EXTENSION WITH TWIST	**12 REPS** *(alternating)*	102

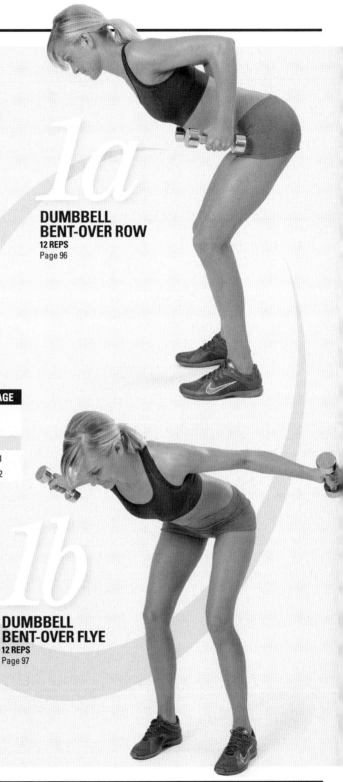

DUMBBELL BENT-OVER ROW
12 REPS
Page 96

REST
40 SECONDS

DUMBBELL BENT-OVER FLYE
12 REPS
Page 97

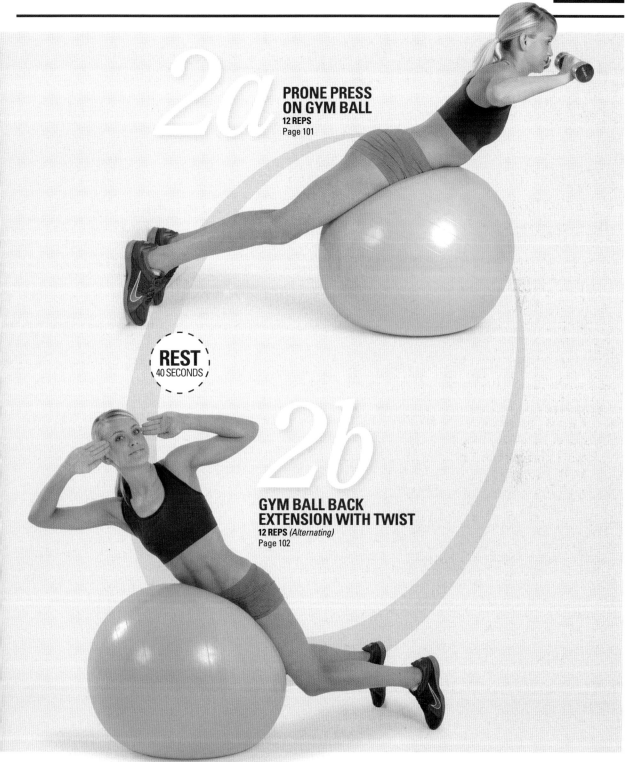

2a

PRONE PRESS ON GYM BALL
12 REPS
Page 101

REST
40 SECONDS

2b

GYM BALL BACK EXTENSION WITH TWIST
12 REPS *(Alternating)*
Page 102

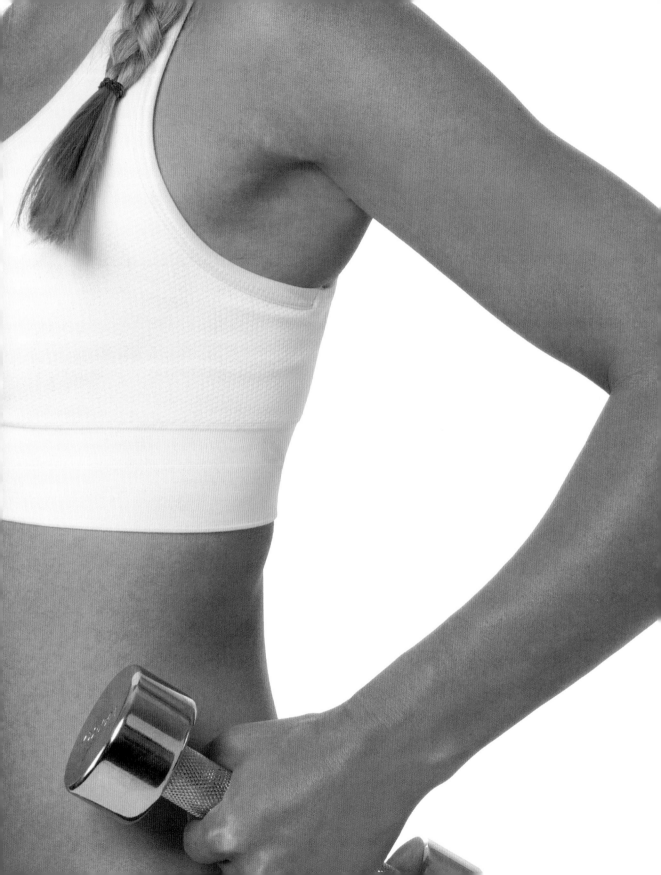

ARMS

There's more to arm workouts than dumbbell curls, you know. Transform your arms into toned, bingo-wing-free zones with these easy moves to challenge triceps, forearms and biceps.

SIX WAYS TO SCULPTED ARMS

1. Doing yoga will tone up your arms fast. In many poses, such as crow, plank and downward-facing dog, your arms are helping support your body weight.

2. Chop and change your swimming stroke to work all parts of your arms. Up the results by wearing webbed gloves or swim with a pull-buoy between your legs.

3. Carry your shopping bags home instead of driving to the supermarket, and use manual appliances instead of labour-saving ones.

4. OK, so they're not always pleasurable, but chores such as gardening, cleaning and DIY are a proper arm workout.

5. Define your upper body tone by having glowing skin. Arms, particularly the backs of them, can be susceptible to bumpy skin, so regularly use a body scrub and loofah mitt to target unevenness.

6. Bring your arms into play while you walk, run and dance. Swinging your arms will increase calorie burn.

EXERCISE ONE

Quick tip!
Don't push your
pelvic area out
as you curl.

RESISTANCE BAND BICEPS CURL

BENEFITS: This move makes your arms work hard at the top of the curl (whereas with dumbbells the tough part's at the bottom).

◆ Stand on a resistance band and grab either end with your hands, keeping a slight bend at the elbow. Your feet should be parallel and shoulder-width apart, your palms facing forwards (*a*).

◆ Keeping your abdominal muscles tight and your elbows tucked in to your sides, curl your hands into your shoulders (*b*).

◆ Return to the start. Aim to do eight to 15 reps.

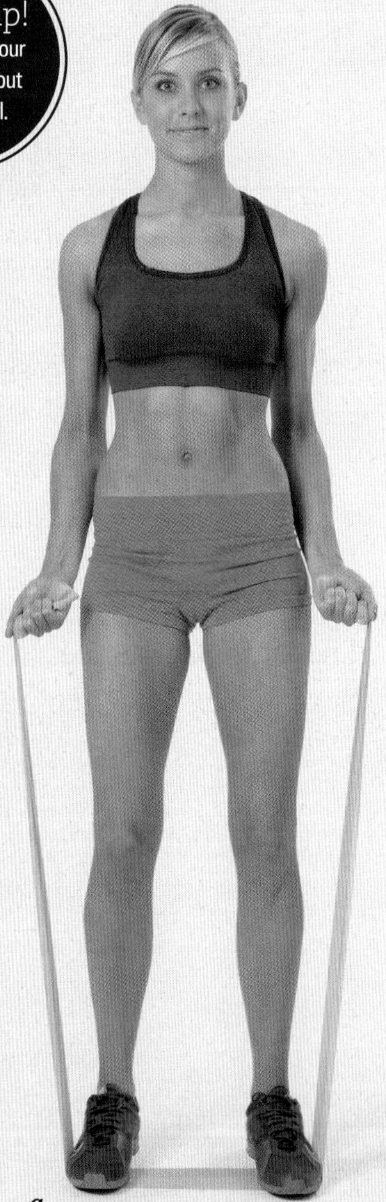

a

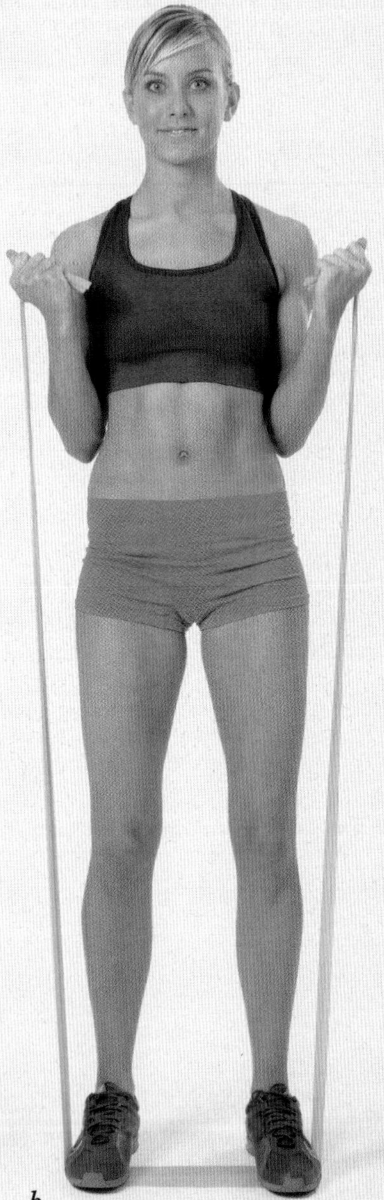

b

EXERCISE TWO

DUMBBELL BENT-OVER TRICEPS KICKBACK

BENEFITS: A fabulous all-over exercise to work your back, triceps, abdominals and legs.

◆ Take your dumbbells and stand, hands by your sides, a dumbbell in each one, palms facing in. Bend from the hips until your torso is parallel to the floor. Bend your knees, making sure they stay over your feet and look down.

◆ Bend your arms and bring your elbows up to shoulder level, keeping them close to your body (*a*).

◆ Hold, then straighten your arms out behind you, squeezing the triceps. Your palms should be facing each other (*b*). Aim to do eight to 15 reps.

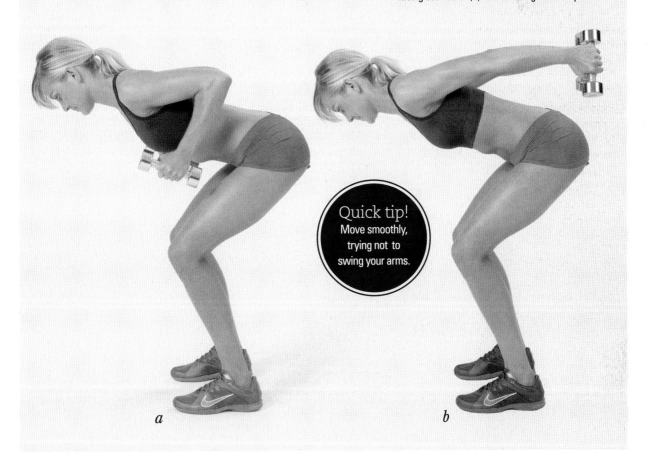

a

b

Quick tip!
Move smoothly, trying not to swing your arms.

EXERCISE THREE

DUMBBELL ZOTTMAN CURL

BENEFITS: A subtle exercise to target all parts of your biceps muscles.

◆ Stand with your spine straight, feet shoulder-width apart and a dumbbell in each hand, palms facing forwards (*a*).

◆ Curl the dumbbells up, keeping your elbows tucked into your sides (*b*).

◆ Rotate your wrists so that your palms face down (*c*), then lower the weights slowly (*d*).

◆ Rotate your wrists again to return to the start position. Aim to do eight to 15 reps.

Quick tip!
Keep your elbows close to your body throughout.

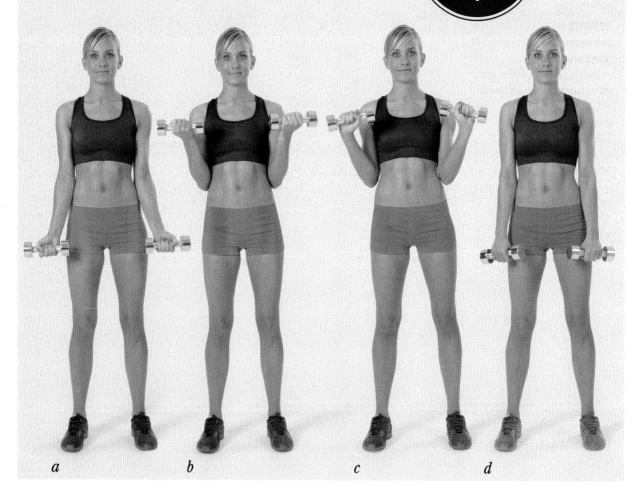

a   *b*   *c*   *d*

EXERCISE FOUR

RESISTANCE BAND TRICEPS EXTENSION

BENEFITS: Great for your back and triceps and for increasing shoulder flexibility.

◆ Place your feet hip-width apart, spine neutral and focus forwards.

◆ Grabbing your resistance band in your right hand, place your hand behind your back then grab the other end of the band with your left hand (*a*).

◆ Extend your right elbow until your arm is fully extended (*b*).

◆ Return to the starting position and aim to repeat six to eight times before swapping sides.

Quick tip!
Don't arch your back as you extend your arms.

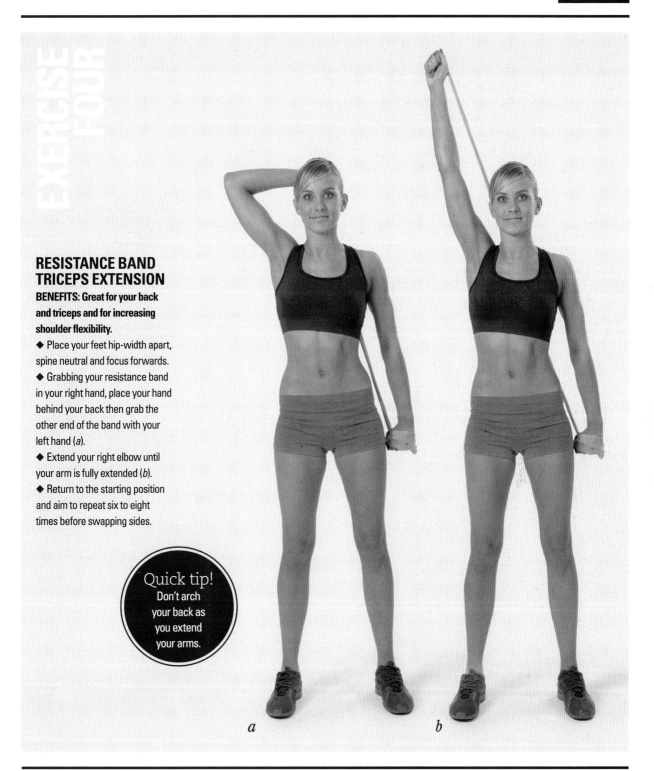

a   *b*

EXERCISE FIVE

DUMBBELL SQUAT TO CURL TO PRESS

BENEFITS: A three-part exercise for your thighs, biceps, shoulders and legs.

◆ Stand with your feet slightly wider than shoulder-width, dumbbells in hands by your sides, palms facing in.

◆ Slowly bend your knees into a squat until your thighs are parallel to the floor. Keep your back straight and feet and knees in line (*a*).

◆ Push through your heels to stand up dynamically, simultaneously curling the dumbbells into your shoulders (*b*).

◆ In another dynamic movement, extend your arms overhead and rotate your hands forwards (*c*).

◆ Return the weights to your shoulders and move back into the squat, then lower your hands to the starting position.
Aim to repeat eight to 15 times.

Quick tip!
Keep your chest open and upright throughout the exercise.

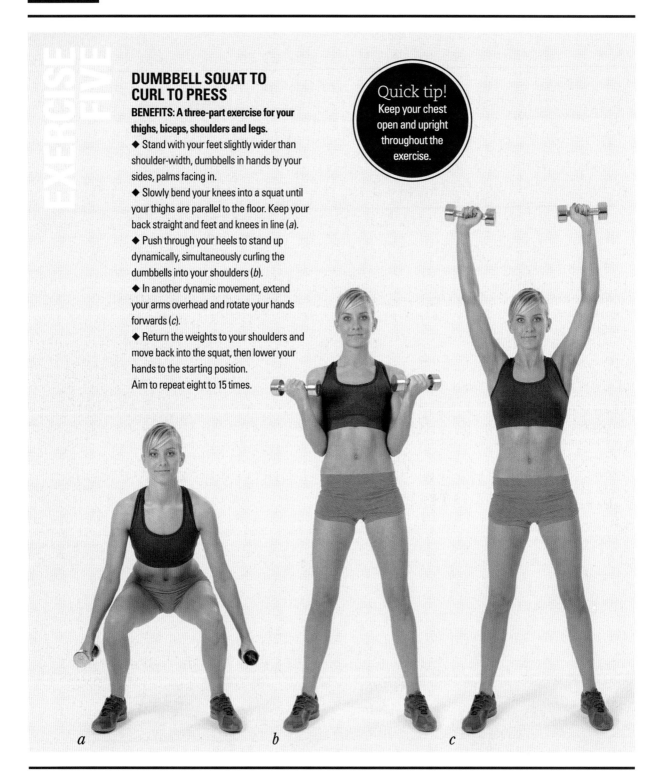

a　　　*b*　　　*c*

EXERCISE SIX

BENT-LEG DIP

BENEFITS: It's another classic move for your shoulders and core as well as your triceps.

◆ Sit on a bench or Step, hands either side of you, fingers pointing forwards and gripping onto the edge.

◆ Step your feet forward and slide your bottom carefully off the bench. Keep your knees bent and your chin parallel to the floor (*a*).

◆ Slowly bend your arms behind you as you lower your bottom (*b*).

◆ Pause, then push yourself up to the straight-arm position. Aim to repeat eight to 15 times.

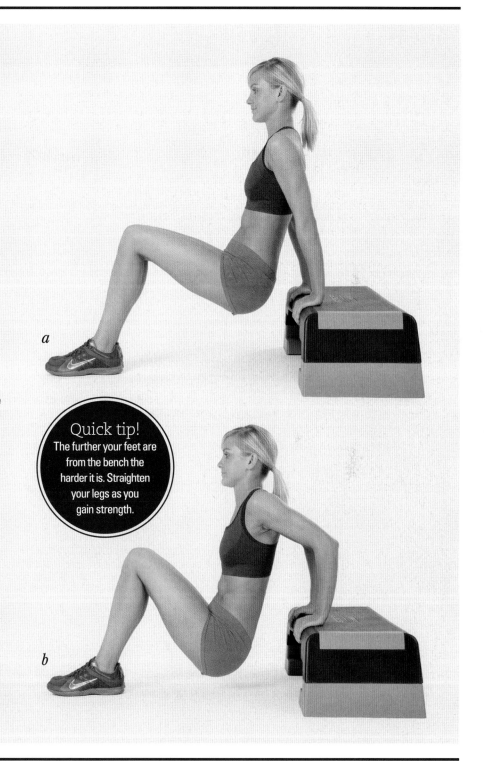

a

b

Quick tip!
The further your feet are from the bench the harder it is. Straighten your legs as you gain strength.

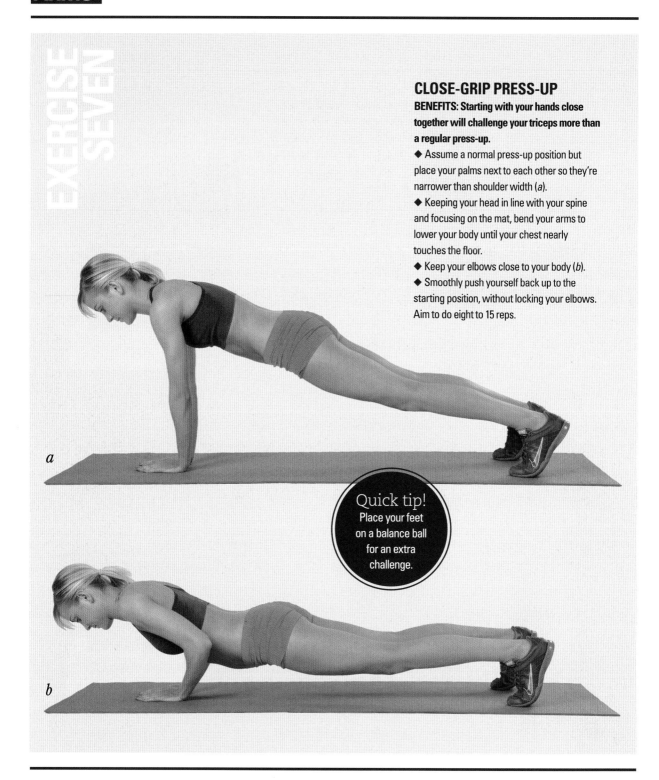

EXERCISE SEVEN

a

b

CLOSE-GRIP PRESS-UP
BENEFITS: Starting with your hands close together will challenge your triceps more than a regular press-up.

◆ Assume a normal press-up position but place your palms next to each other so they're narrower than shoulder width (*a*).

◆ Keeping your head in line with your spine and focusing on the mat, bend your arms to lower your body until your chest nearly touches the floor.

◆ Keep your elbows close to your body (*b*).

◆ Smoothly push yourself back up to the starting position, without locking your elbows. Aim to do eight to 15 reps.

Quick tip!
Place your feet on a balance ball for an extra challenge.

EXERCISE EIGHT

CUBAN PRESS

BENEFITS: Tests all parts of your arms and shoulders, and great for increasing your range of movement.

◆ Stand with your feet shoulder-width apart, dumbbells resting on your upper thighs, palms facing backwards (*a*).

◆ Raise your elbows until your upper arms are in line with your shoulders. Your palms should still be facing backwards, and keep a 90° angle between your upper arms and forearms (*b*).

◆ Rotate your elbows, raising the dumbbells so your palms are now facing forwards. Your upper arms should still be in line with your shoulders, and maintain the 90° bend in your elbows (*c*).

◆ Keeping your lower body still, raise your arms into a press, hands above shoulders, palms still facing forwards, keeping a slight bend in your elbows (*d*).

◆ Reverse through the stages to return to the start. Aim to do eight to 15 reps.

Quick tip!
Avoid hunching your shoulders as you move through the stages of the exercise.

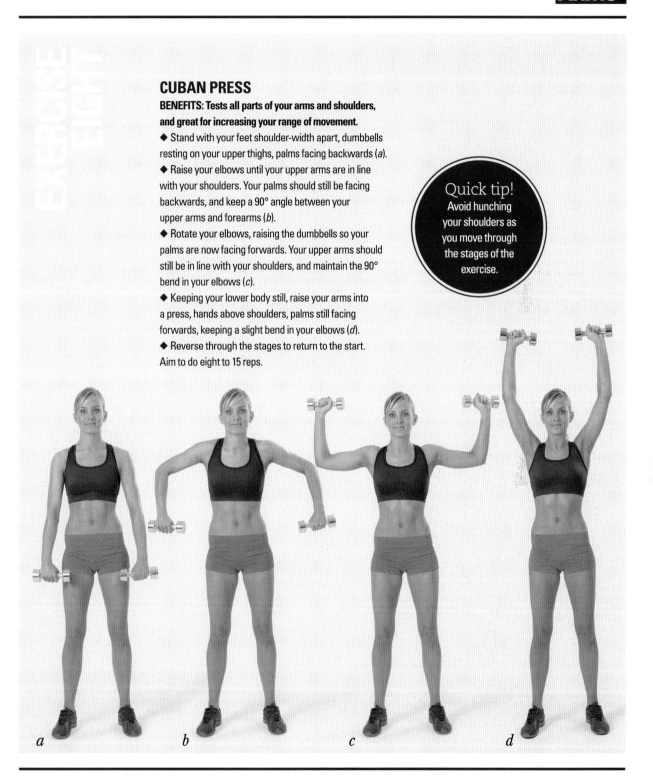

a　　　　*b*　　　　*c*　　　　*d*

10-MINUTE ARMS WORKOUT
BEGINNER

Beginners should arm themselves with this simple circuit.

WHAT TO DO… Grab and prepare your resistance band. Do a thorough warm-up, then perform this circuit three times. Rest for 30 seconds between exercises 2 and 3 and for 30 seconds between circuits.

EXERCISES	REPS/DURATION	PAGE
1. LUNGE TO FLYE	30 SECONDS *(alternating)*	17
2. RESISTANCE BAND BICEPS CURL	12 REPS	112
REST	30 SECONDS	
3. JUMPING JACKS	30 SECONDS	17
4. RESISTANCE BAND TRICEPS EXTENSION	12 REPS *(each side)*	115
REST	30 SECONDS	

1
LUNGE TO FLYE
30 SECONDS *(alternating)*
Page 17

REST
30 SECONDS

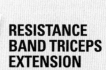

4
RESISTANCE BAND TRICEPS EXTENSION
12 REPS *(each side)*
Page 115

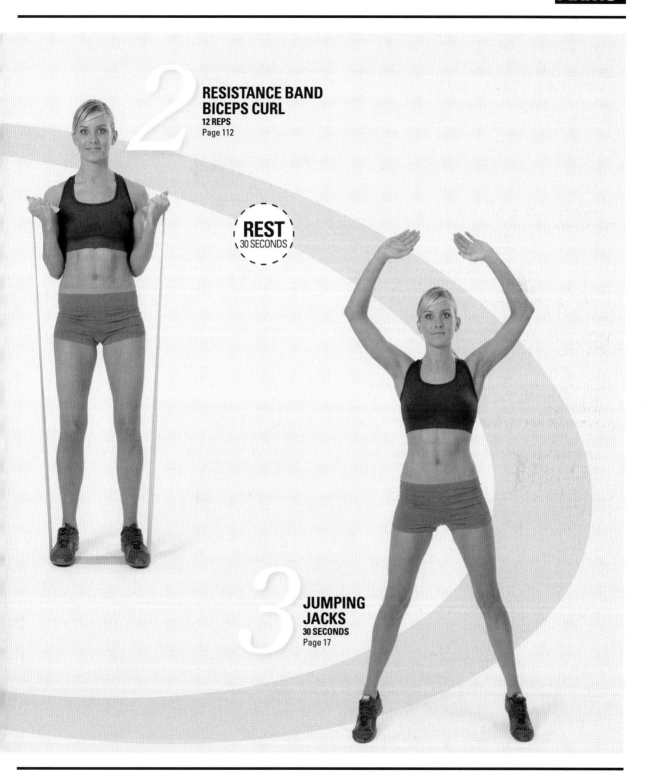

2

RESISTANCE BAND
BICEPS CURL
12 REPS
Page 112

REST
30 SECONDS

3

JUMPING
JACKS
30 SECONDS
Page 17

10-MINUTE ARMS WORKOUT
INTERMEDIATE

A duo of arm supersets for intermediates.

WHAT TO DO… Do exercise 1a followed immediately by exercise 1b – that's one superset. Perform superset 1 three times, resting for 30 seconds between each set. Then rest for one minute before moving on to do the same with superset 2.

EXERCISES	REPS/DURATION	PAGE
1a. DUMBBELL ZOTTMAN CURL	12 REPS	114
1b. DUMBBELL BENT-OVER TRICEPS KICKBACK	10 REPS	113
REST	1 MINUTE	
2a. BENT-LEG DIP	10 REPS	117
2b. CUBAN PRESS	10 REPS	119

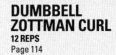

1a
DUMBBELL ZOTTMAN CURL
12 REPS
Page 114

REST
30 SECONDS

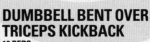

1b
DUMBBELL BENT OVER TRICEPS KICKBACK
10 REPS
Page 113

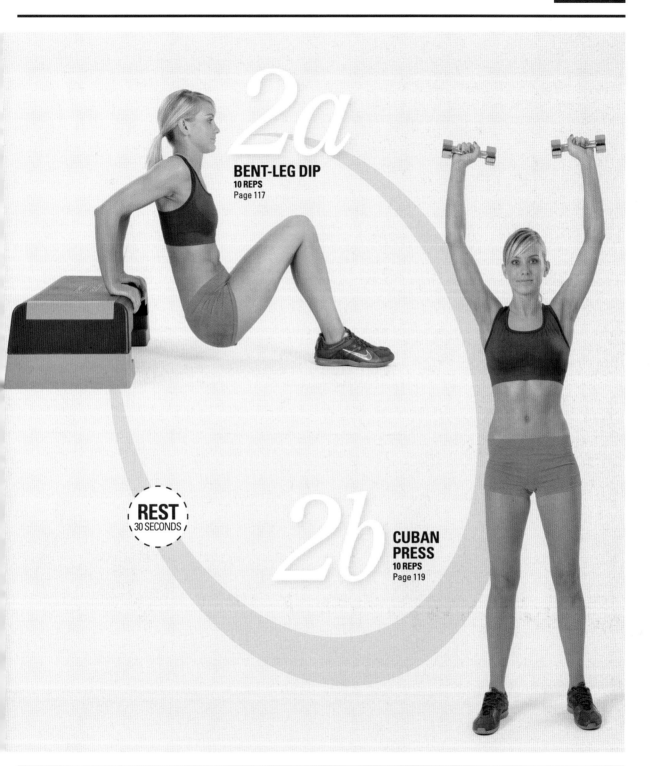

2a

BENT-LEG DIP
10 REPS
Page 117

REST
30 SECONDS

2b

CUBAN
PRESS
10 REPS
Page 119

10-MINUTE ARMS WORKOUT
ADVANCED

An advanced arm circuit for the experienced.

WHAT TO DO… Do a full warm-up and repeat this circuit three times, resting for 30 seconds between each circuit. Make sure your dumbbells and Step or bench are prepared in advance.

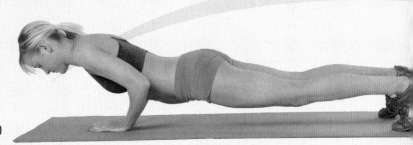

1

CLOSE-GRIP PRESS-UP
10 REPS *(or as many as you can)*
Page 118

EXERCISES	REPS/DURATION	PAGE
1. CLOSE-GRIP PRESS-UP	**10 REPS** *(or max)*	118
2. DUMBBELL SQUAT TO CURL TO PRESS	**10 REPS**	116
3. STRAIGHT-LEG DIP	**10 REPS** *(or max)*	117
4. DUMBBELL SQUAT TO CURL TO PRESS	**10 REPS**	116
5. DUMBBELL BENT-OVER TRICEPS KICKBACK	**10 REPS**	113
6. DUMBBELL SQUAT TO CURL TO PRESS	**10 REPS**	116
REST	30 SECONDS	

REST
30 SECONDS

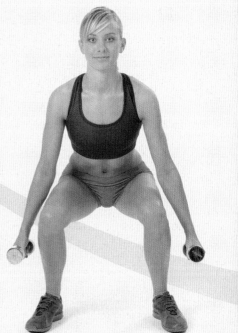

6

DUMBBELL SQUAT TO CURL TO PRESS
10 REPS
Page 116

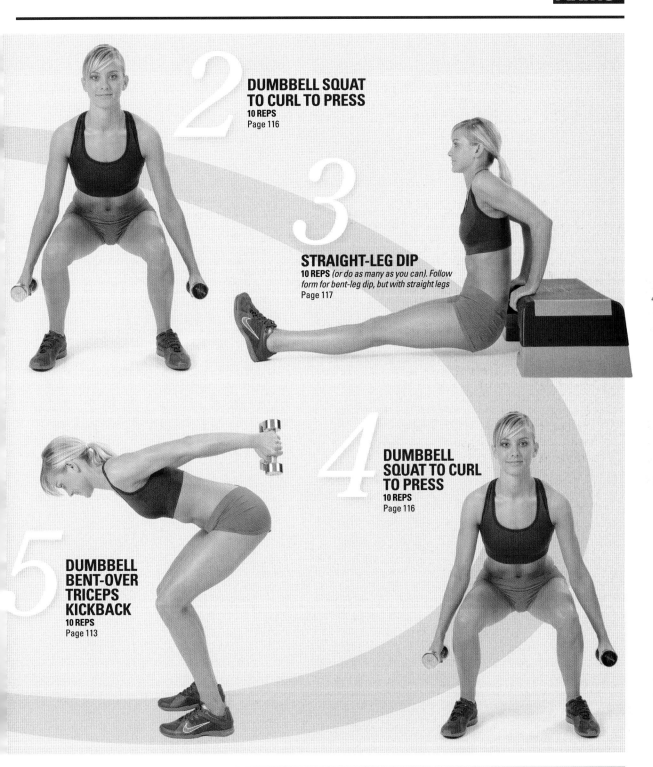

2
DUMBBELL SQUAT TO CURL TO PRESS
10 REPS
Page 116

3
STRAIGHT-LEG DIP
10 REPS *(or do as many as you can). Follow form for bent-leg dip, but with straight legs*
Page 117

4
DUMBBELL SQUAT TO CURL TO PRESS
10 REPS
Page 116

5
DUMBBELL BENT-OVER TRICEPS KICKBACK
10 REPS
Page 113

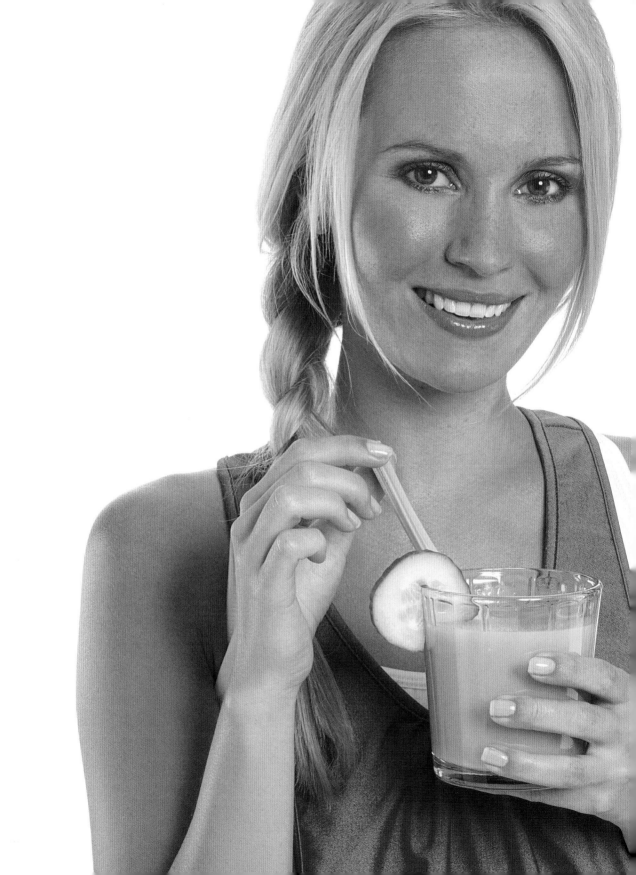

DIET

There's no point doing endless tummy-toning exercises then not seeing the benefits because you're eating all the wrong foods. The following pages contain expert advice on healthy eating, plus a simple seven-day menu plan and some inspiring nutritious recipe ideas.

SIX WAYS TO BEAT THE BLOAT

1. Hold the salt. Water is attracted to sodium, so when you eat salty foods you retain fluid, leading to bloating and puffiness.
2. Avoid gassy foods. Some foods create more wind in your digestive tract than others. These include beans and pulses, cauliflower, broccoli, Brussels sprouts, cabbage, onions, peppers and citrus fruits.
3. Don't chew gum. While you chew, you swallow air, which gets trapped and causes bloating.
4. Cut down on fried foods. Fatty foods, especially fried ones, are digested more slowly, causing you to feel heavy and bloated.
5. Skip spicy foods. Seasonings such as black pepper, chilli powder, hot sauces, onions, garlic and fresh chillies can speed up food transit time in the gut which encourages wind.
6. No more fizzy drinks. Those bubbles can cause excess air in your digestive system.

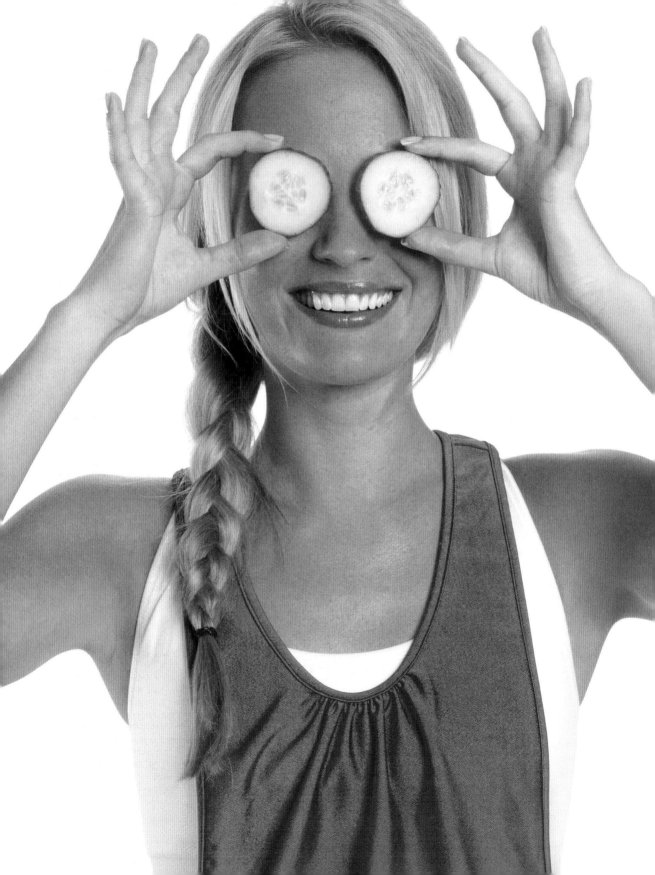

EAT SLIM!

Combine your workouts with these healthy eating tips to stay slim and healthy for life.

Whether you want a flat stomach and firm bottom, or you need to lose a few pounds to fit into that favourite dress, the key to success is to combine exercise with a healthy diet. There's no point doing endless tummy-toning exercises if your abdominals are hidden under a layer of calorie-induced flab!

Experts agree the best way to lose weight is slowly and steadily. A weight loss of 1–2lb (0.5–1kg) a week is ideal. Studies show people who lose weight this way are much more likely keep the weight off.

To lose 1lb of fat a week you need to lose roughly 500 calories a day. You can do this by reducing the number of calories you eat or by increasing the amount of calories you burn. But the easiest and best way is a combination of diet and exercise. Think of a Mars bar – it takes two minutes to eat but about 30 minutes of running to burn off the calories! Combine exercise with healthy eating, and the results can be amazing.

If you want to follow a structured weight-loss diet, turn the page to find our nutritious four-week superfood plan. Or, for a less structured approach, follow our six daily healthy eating rules to stay slim and healthy for life.

1 **Always eat breakfast.** You've heard it a million times before, but eating breakfast is vital for keeping you slim. When you wake up, your blood-sugar levels are low as your body's been fasting all night. A good breakfast, combining protein and carbohydrate (for instance porridge with nuts and seeds) will stop you snacking later on, and ensure you have the energy to get going.

2 **Eat three meals a day along with a healthy, low-fat snack, morning and afternoon.** This will help keep your blood sugar levels constant, avoiding excess hunger or cravings that can make you want to fill up on the first high-fat, sugary food you can get your hands on.

3 **Choose natural wholesome, foods as often as possible.** Swap white bread, pasta and rice for low-GI wholegrain varieties that contain more fibre to keep you fuller for longer. Ditch processed foods and convenience meals, often high in unhealthy fats, and instead eat plenty of oily fish (rich in healthy fats), lean meat, fruit and vegetables. Including a variety of nutrient-dense foods in your diet will fill you up on fewer calories and ensure you get all the nutrients you need.

4 **Include protein at every meal.** Your body has to work hard to digest protein and this helps boost your metabolic rate and burn calories. Try to include some lean protein in every meal and snack. Good choices include lean meat, fish, eggs, beans, pulses, cheese, milk, nuts and seeds.

5 **Control your portions.** Eating the right foods is only half the story when it comes to weight loss. Eating the right amount of food is just as important. A meat serving should be the size of a pack of cards, a pasta portion as big as your fist and a serving of cheese the size of a matchbox. Try serving your food on smaller plates and eating slowly to ensure you don't eat more than you need.

6 **Drink at least eight glasses of water a day**. Not only is this essential to keep you hydrated and healthy, it will help keep you feeling full and beat water retention. It's easy to confuse hunger with thirst and eat when what you really need is fluid. Make sure you drink extra water when you're exercising or in hot weather, to compensate for sweat loss and help you perform at your best.

FUEL UP!

Eat the right foods at the right times to boost your workouts and recover quickly

You need to start out with a 'full tank' to ensure you perform at your best and avoid fatigue when exercising. Eating (even if it's a healthy snack) every four hours is vital for active people.

If you're exercising early in the morning, have a glass of juice or a banana before – and don't skip breakfast after. If you're exercising later in the day, have a snack about an hour before your workout, such as a banana, muesli bar, handful of dried fruit or a smoothie. Drink plenty of water before and after your workouts.

After your workout, you must rehydrate with water, then refuel, so eat a healthy meal after. If your workout has lasted more than an hour, eat a healthy snack within half an hour of finishing to replenish your muscles' glycogen stores. Try a banana smoothie, a bowl of cereal or a couple of slices of toast.

DIET PLAN

Lose pounds and look your best with our superfood diet plan.

How the plan works

Packed with nutritious superfoods, this four-week weight-loss plan will keep you healthy as well as slim. Designed to help you lose at least half a stone when combined with exercise, it will have you looking in great shape in a month's time.

The diet plan is based on 1,500 calories a day. You can have around 300 calories for breakfast, 400 calories for lunch and 600 calories for dinner, plus a piece of fruit or low-fat yoghurt mid-morning and afternoon. Simply select one choice from the breakfast, lunch and dinner suggestions. You're also allowed 200ml semi-skimmed milk for tea or coffee. All recipe suggestions are for one.

10 TOP SUPERFOODS

These inexpensive, everyday foods can easily be included in your diet – but the benefits they offer are anything but ordinary

Oily fish Fish such as sardines, fresh tuna and mackerel are rich in omega 3 fatty acids that can reduce risk of heart attack and stroke, as well as keep your skin glowing.

Broccoli An excellent source of vitamins A and C and folic acid, broccoli contains phytochemicals believed to protect against cancer.

Soya In countries where soya and soya products are eaten regularly, heart disease, breast cancer and osteoporosis are less common. Eating 25g soya protein a day will help reduce cholesterol. Try tofu or soya milk.

Probiotic yoghurts These maintain good bacteria in your gut that help strengthen your immunity and digestion. One pot of yoghurt provides almost a quarter of your daily calcium needs.

Red peppers An excellent source of vitamin C, red peppers contain over twice as much vitamin C as oranges.

Berries All varieties contain antioxidant polyphenols, which are thought to help prevent cancers. They also soothe inflammation in the body, so they're great for helping you recover from intense exercise.

Sweet potatoes These vegetables contain more vitamin E than any other low-fat food. They're also an excellent source of betacarotene, vitamin C, potassium and vitamin B6.

Nuts and seeds These are packed with protein, vitamins, minerals and essential brain-enhancing and immune-boosting fatty acids.

Oats The soluble fibre in oats lowers cholesterol and helps stabilise blood sugar levels, reducing risk of coronary heart disease and type II diabetes.

Beans The fibre in beans lowers cholesterol, combats heart disease and cancer, stabilises blood sugar and lowers blood pressure.

Breakfast
(300 calories)

DAY ONE

Banoffee smoothie Blend 150ml low-fat vanilla yoghurt, 200ml skimmed milk, 1 small sliced banana and 1 tbsp maple syrup until smooth. Plus eat 1 slice of granary toast or 1 low-fat cereal bar.

DAY TWO

Apple and blackberry smoothie Blend 300ml apple juice and 125g frozen blackberries until smooth. Plus eat 1 slice of granary toast or 1 low-fat cereal bar.

DAY THREE

Mango and melon smoothie Blend the flesh of 1 ripe mango and half a Galia melon with 200ml apple juice until smooth. Plus eat 1 slice of granary toast or 1 low-fat cereal bar.

DAY FOUR

Figs with ricotta Mix 50g ricotta cheese with 1 tsp icing sugar and zest of 1 orange. Spread over 1 thick slice (about 40g) of granary toast. Top with 1 thickly sliced fresh fig. Plus drink 150ml cranberry juice.

DAY FIVE

Lemon and raspberry muesli Stir 2 tbsp of sugar-free muesli, the zest of ½ lemon and 50g fresh raspberries into 200ml low-fat yoghurt. Plus drink 150ml cranberry juice.

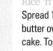

DAY SIX

Rice 'n' peanuts Spread 1 tbsp of peanut butter over 1 large rice cake. Top with 1 small sliced banana. Plus drink 150ml fruit juice.

DAY SEVEN

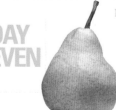

Eggs too easy Top 1 thick slice of granary toast with 1 poached or boiled egg. Plus drink 150ml fruit juice and eat 1 pear.

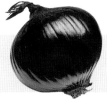

Lunch
(400 calories)

For lunch and dinner, choose one suggestion from the list plus a piece of fruit, a fruit salad or a low-fat yoghurt.

Red pepper houmous Slice 1 small red pepper in half and grill for 15 minutes. Peel off the skin and roughly chop the flesh. Stir into 50g reduced-fat houmous. Serve with 1 wholemeal pitta and a handful of cherry tomatoes.

Quick gazpacho Blend a 330ml can V8 juice, ½ small red pepper, ½ small red onion, ½ cucumber, 1 clove of garlic, a pinch of sugar and 1 tsp olive oil until smooth. Serve with a hunk (about 50g) of granary bread.

Mixed-bean salad Mix 4 tbsp of canned mixed beans with 2 finely chopped spring onions and ½ diced red pepper, 100g tuna in brine (drained) and 1 tbsp French dressing.

Charred asparagus with a poached egg Cook 6 spears of asparagus until just tender. Toast 1 thick slice of granary bread and top with the asparagus and a poached egg.

Prawn fajita wrap Heat 1 tsp oil in a non-stick frying pan, add 75g cooked prawns, 2 finely chopped spring onions and 1 tsp fajita seasoning and stir-fry for 1 minute. Heat 1 small soft flour tortilla, spoon in the prawns and 2 halved cherry tomatoes and ½ small sliced avocado.

Chicken and mango salad Mix 1 tbsp reduced-fat mayonnaise, 1 tbsp plain low-fat yoghurt, 1 tbsp mango chutney, 1 tsp mild curry paste and stir the mixture in to 75g cooked brown rice. Add 2 finely chopped spring onions, 1 chopped stick of celery, ½ diced mango and 1 small skinless chicken breast.

Pea and ham frittata Whisk 2 eggs with 4 tbsp skimmed milk and season. Stir in 50g cooked frozen peas and 50g chopped smoked ham. Heat 2 tsp vegetable oil in a pan and pour in the egg mixture. Cook over a low heat for 4–5 minutes or until the bottom is just set. Place under a pre-heated grill and cook for a further 4–5 minutes or until just firm to the touch. Serve with a green salad with low-fat dressing.

Dinner
(600 calories)

Chicken with sweet and sour onions Heat 1 tbsp olive oil in a pan, add 1 sliced red onion and cook over a gentle heat for 10–15 minutes. Add 1 tbsp balsamic vinegar, 1 tbsp sugar, 1 tbsp raisins and 1 tsp pine nuts and cook for 5 minutes. Place 1 chicken escalope on a hot griddle pan and cook for a couple of minutes either side. Pile the onions on to a plate and top with the chicken. Serve with a baked sweet potato.

Vietnamese tuna salad Pour boiling water over a sheet of dried egg noodles and leave to stand for 5 minutes. Mix 1 tbsp soy sauce, 2 tsp sesame oil and 1 crushed clove of garlic and rub over 1 small (125g) tuna steak. Place the tuna on a hot griddle pan and cook for 2–3 minutes either side. Drain the noodles and mix with a handful of green salad leaves. Mix the juice of 1 lime with 1 tbsp sweet chilli sauce and drizzle over the salad. Top with the tuna.

Spaghetti with fresh tomatoes and parsley Cook 50g wholemeal spaghetti until just tender. Remove the skin and seeds from 4 plum tomatoes and slice the flesh into small cubes. Drain the pasta, stir in the tomatoes, 6 roughly chopped pitted black olives, 2 tbsp of chopped fresh parsley, the zest of 1 lemon and 1 tbsp of olive oil.

Vegetable kebabs with couscous and mint dressing Place 50g quick-cook couscous and 1–2 strands of saffron in a bowl and pour over 125ml vegetable stock. Leave to stand for 15 minutes. Stir in 2 chopped spring onions and 1 tbsp sultanas. Thread a selection of vegetables on to a skewer. Brush with olive oil, place on a hot griddle pan and cook, turning occasionally, for 5–6 minutes or until tender. Mix 4 tbsp low-fat natural bio yoghurt with 1 tsp mint sauce. Serve the kebabs on couscous with dressing.

Teriyaki chicken with shiitake mushrooms Slice 1 skinless chicken breast into thin strips and marinate in 2 tbsp of teriyaki sauce for 10 minutes. Heat 2 tsp of oil in a wok, add the chicken and stir-fry for 3–4 minutes. Add 3 thinly sliced spring onions, 1 crushed clove of garlic and 100g roughly chopped shiitake mushrooms and cook until tender. Serve with 100g cooked brown rice.

Spanish eggs Heat 2 tsp of olive oil in a non-stick pan, add 1 small finely chopped onion and 1 crushed clove of garlic and cook for 2–3 minutes. Add a 400g can of chopped tomatoes, a pinch of sugar, smoked paprika and ground cumin and cook for 15 minutes. Spoon the mixture into a shallow oven-proof dish. Crack 2 omega-3-enriched eggs into the tomato mixture and transfer to a hot oven, 200°C/gas mark 6 for 10–15 minutes. Serve with tenderstem broccoli and a thick slice (50g) of granary bread.

Maple and mustard glazed salmon Mix 1 tbsp wholegrain mustard and 1 tbsp maple syrup. Place 1 salmon fillet (about 125g) skin-side down on a shallow ovenproof tray and spread with the maple syrup mixture. Grill for 10 minutes or until cooked through. Serve with steamed asparagus and 3 small new potatoes.

RECIPES

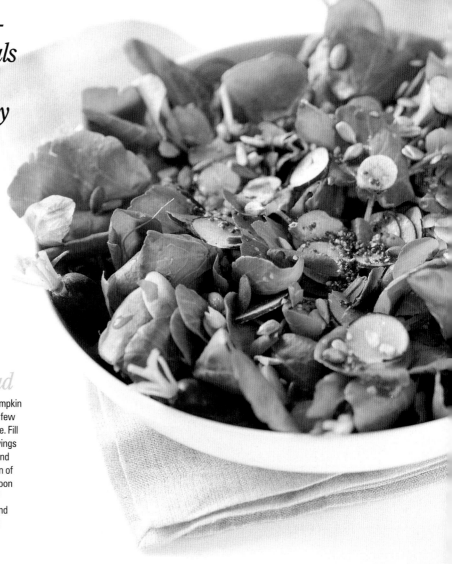

Rustling up tasty – and healthy – meals doesn't have to be a chore. These easy recipes have all the nutrients your hardworking body needs.

Watercress, radish and toasted seed salad

Add a dessertspoon each of sunflower and pumpkin seeds to a dry frying pan and cook gently for a few minutes until they start to brown, then set aside. Fill a bowl with watercress and sprinkle with shavings of radish, arranging a few whole radishes around the bowl. Make a dressing with one tablespoon of extra-virgin olive oil mixed with one dessertspoon of freshly-squeezed lemon juice, a teaspoon of wholegrain mustard and a pinch each of salt and pepper. Drizzle the dressing over the salad and sprinkle with seeds. Serves two to three.

Minted pea soup

Soups are brilliant for getting a few of your five-a-day. To make this fresh, summer variety, soften a small, finely chopped onion in a little sunflower oil, but don't let the onion brown. Add 150g peeled, diced potato and 500ml vegetable stock. Simmer for 10 to 12 minutes until the potato is soft, then add 250g fresh or frozen peas and 6 to 10 fresh mint leaves. Return to the boil, remove from the heat and blend. Taste and season with salt and pepper. Serve hot or cold with a blob of crème fraîche or Greek yoghurt and a sprig of fresh mint.

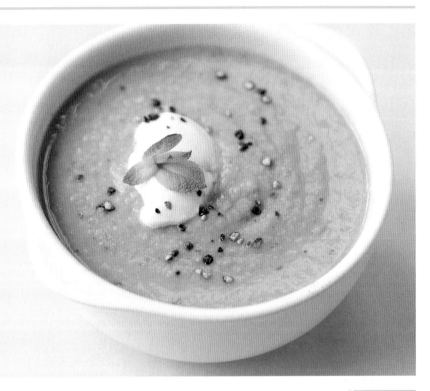

Wholemeal pasta with pea and walnut pesto

In a hot pan, soften a finely chopped onion in a dash of olive oil. Add 75g peas (fresh or defrosted frozen) and 20g walnut pieces and mix. Blend a further 75g peas and 20g walnuts, clove of garlic, handful each of parsley and basil, sprigs of mint, 1 tbsp natural yoghurt, 1 tsp walnut oil, and salt and pepper. Mix this pesto and the contents of the pan with 250g cooked wholemeal pasta and serve.

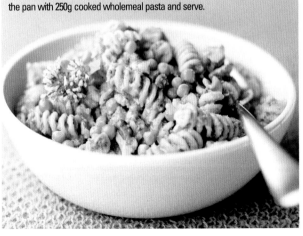

Muesli bars

Mash 2 bananas and mix with an unpeeled apple roughly chopped into cubes, 2 cups rolled oats, 1 cup apple juice, ½ cup of mixed dried fruit, ½ cup of chopped apricots and 1 tsp each of sunflower seeds, pumpkin seeds and linseeds. Spread the mixture out on a baking sheet so it's 2cm thick. Press a few whole apricots into the top. Bake for 15–20 minutes in a medium oven, 180°C/gas mark 4. Allow it to cool a little, then cut into bars and serve.

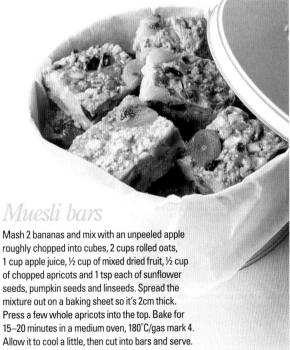

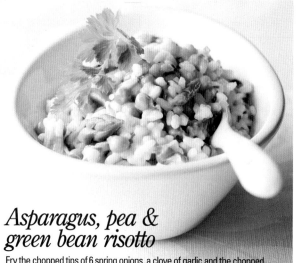

Asparagus, pea & green bean risotto

Fry the chopped tips of 6 spring onions, a clove of garlic and the chopped stems of a bunch of asparagus in olive oil. Add 200g risotto rice, season and stir. Add a glass of white wine, allow to evaporate, then stir in 750ml hot organic chicken or vegetable stock. With the stock, stir in 100g green beans, 150g peas, stems of the spring onions and the asparagus tips. When the stock is absorbed, after 10–12 minutes, add chopped parsley and 1 tbsp crème fraîche, stir and serve.

Kiwifruit, pear and apple smoothie

Kiwifruit are packed with potassium, antioxidants, fibre and vitamins C and E. To make this delicious smoothie, peel 2 ripe kiwifruit, then peel and core 1 large ripe pear and blend together with a 1 cup cloudy apple juice. Simply add the ingredients to a large jug and blend together with a hand-held blender until smooth. By pulping whole fruit you capture the maximum number of nutrients.

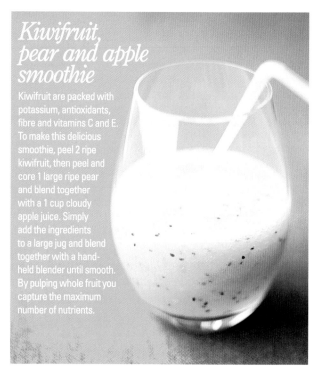

Chargrilled fennel with salmon

Top and tail a bulb of fennel, then cut into wedges. Plunge into a pan of boiling water for a couple of minutes and drain. Meanwhile, place 2 slices of salmon into a hot frying pan with a dash of oil. Cook skin-side down for 4 to 5 minutes. Turn the fish over, add 12 cherry tomatoes and cook for a further 3 minutes. Remove from the heat and leave to rest. While the fish rests, add the fennel to a very hot griddle pan and cook for 4 to 5 minutes, turning a couple of times. Divide the fennel between two plates and add a piece of salmon, some cherry tomatoes and six black olives to each plate. Drizzle with lemon juice, a little extra-virgin olive oil and black pepper, then add a sprig of dill. Can also be served as a cold salad by breaking the salmon into large flakes and arranging everything on a platter.

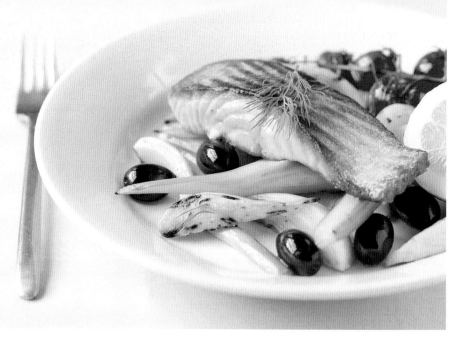

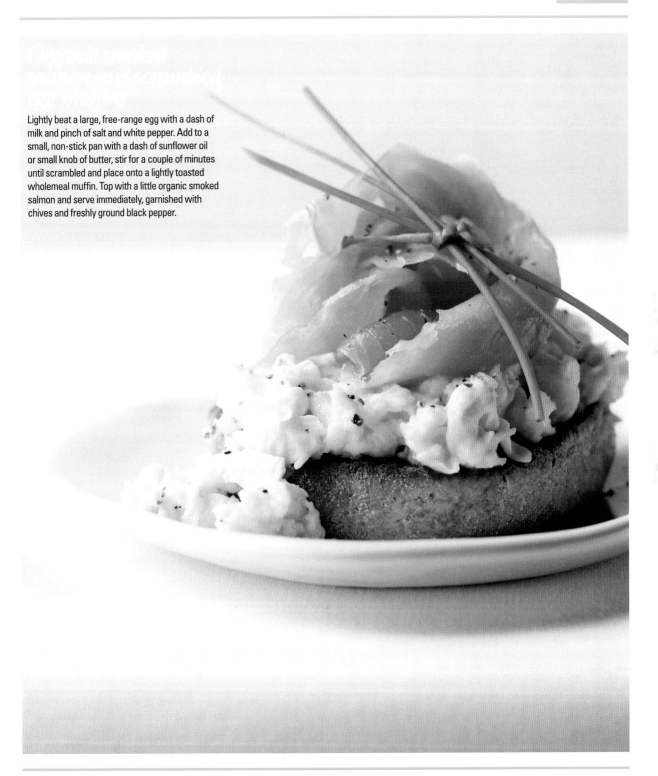

Lightly beat a large, free-range egg with a dash of milk and pinch of salt and white pepper. Add to a small, non-stick pan with a dash of sunflower oil or small knob of butter, stir for a couple of minutes until scrambled and place onto a lightly toasted wholemeal muffin. Top with a little organic smoked salmon and serve immediately, garnished with chives and freshly ground black pepper.

GET SLIM & FIT, FAST

WITH YOUR BEGINNER'S GUIDE TO RUNNING

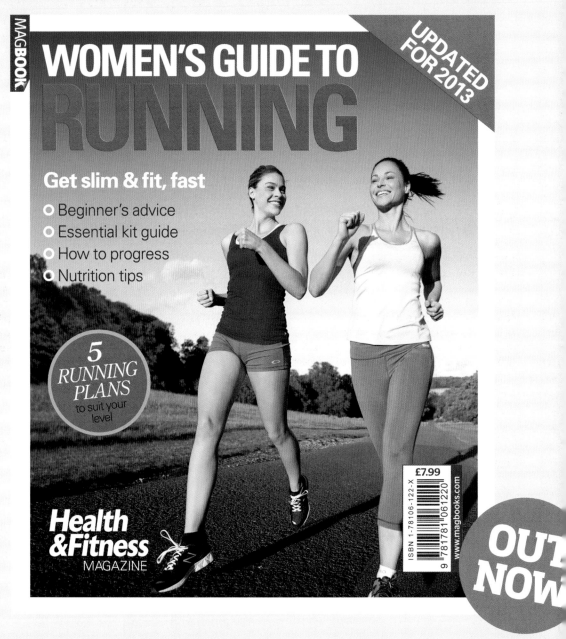

MAGBOOK

WOMEN'S GUIDE TO RUNNING

UPDATED FOR 2013

Get slim & fit, fast

- Beginner's advice
- Essential kit guide
- How to progress
- Nutrition tips

5 RUNNING PLANS
to suit your level

Health &Fitness MAGAZINE

£7.99

ISBN 1-78106-122-X

www.magbooks.com

9 781781 061220

OUT NOW

Order your print or digital MagBook
at magbooks.com

Track your PROGRESS

This is the place to monitor your results. Record your vital statistics before you begin your workout plan and test yourself every four weeks to monitor your progress. Feel free to include your own tests, for instance body fat or the time it takes you to run a particular distance.

To know where you're heading you need to know where you're coming from. Before embarking on your new programme, measure and record four key areas of your fitness – body shape, aerobic capacity, strength and flexibility – in the chart below. Repeat the measurements every four weeks. For continuity's sake, always complete these DIY tests in the same environment.

YOUR FLEXIBILITY
To test your lower back and hamstring flexibility, sit on the floor with your spine straight and legs extended. Bend from the hips (don't curve your spine) and see how far you can extend your fingers down your legs. Make a note of your result.

YOUR SHAPE
Bypass scales – the circumference of key areas such as your hips, waist and thighs is a better gauge of weight loss and tone. Measure your bust, just above the nipple line; your waist, around your belly button; your thigh, about a quarter of the way down; and your bottom, at its widest point.

YOUR AEROBIC FITNESS
Measure your resting heart rate, by feeling your pulse on your wrist or neck (count for six seconds then multiply by 10) or use a monitor if you have one handy. Then complete a step test: simply step up and down, maintaining a steady rhythm for three minutes. Record your heart rate again. As the weeks progress it will decrease and return more quickly to its resting rate.

YOUR STRENGTH
Count how many press-ups you can complete with good form in a minute. If you're a complete beginner, perform them with your knees in contact with the mat until you're stronger. For a whole-body perspective, also do minute tests for sit-ups and squats.

PROGRESS CHART

	Week 1	Week 4	Week 8	Week 12
FLEXIBILITY				
BUST				
WAIST				
THIGHS				
BOTTOM				
RESTING PULSE				
STEP TEST				
PRESS-UP				
SIT-UP				
SQUAT				

Take some 'me time' with *Health & Fitness*

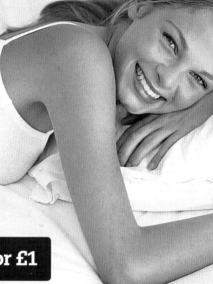

Kick back with *Health & Fitness* magazine and learn all there is to know about toning up, staying healthy and getting fit.

Subscribe and get 3 issues for £1

ORDER ONLINE AT
dennismags.co.uk/healthandfitness
Call 0844 499 1763
using offer code G1301PM